Medicine in Three Societies

Medicine in Three Societies

By Doctor John Fry

*A comparison of medical
care in the USSR, USA and UK*

Published by MTP
Chiltern House
Aylesbury Bucks

ACKNOWLEDGEMENTS

The Milbank Memorial Fund of New York
and the World Health Organisation are
thanked for making my visits possible. To
Dr. Alexander 'Sandy' Robertson of Milbank
and Dr. R.F. Bridgman of WHO, I owe special
thanks.
Dr. Victor Sidel of Boston, U.S.A., was of great
help in the early stages.
Dr. T.M. Ryan and Gordon McLachlan read
through the drafts and made helpful sugges-
tions.
Mrs. K. Sabel did the typing of the many
drafts, and I thank her most sincerely.

Printed in Great Britain by
Billing & Sons Limited
Guildford and London

Contents

Preface and Introduction

This book is a personal testimony of faith in the future and in the progression to better health and a better life. It is the testament of a rough and ready measuring device – a practising physician who sought to compare and contrast three systems of medical care to see what can be distilled from them to help us all in achieving better services for medical care.

Medical care as a human and civic right is the concern of us all. Seeking to live longer and in good health we depend on medical, social and welfare services to attain this goal. Yet it is quite obvious that there are limits and dilemmas that prevent anything but an unsatisfactory compromise. The resources that are available cannot meet all the calls. How then can we make the best use of the resources that we have? This must be the theme for this book. What can we learn from each other for the common good? Since we all are facing the same common problems, how do we go about resolving them? For example, how do the medical care services in the USSR, USA and UK cope with an acute heart attack, with a middle-aged woman with depression, with a brain-damaged child, with a road accident or with a case of measles? These are the common human factors involved.

What is the 'best-buy' in medical care? Is there a system that is superior to all others that can be copied, adapted and reinforced to match local and national patterns?

These and many other questions were in my head when as a working British general practitioner I had the opportunities to visit the USA in 1965/66 and the USSR in 1967. The two months spent in the USA were as a Milbank Memorial Fund Fellow and the five weeks in the USSR were as a consultant to a World Health Organisation Seminar on the 'Organisation of Medical Care'. In both countries I was able and encouraged to visit and study all levels and forms of medical care services.

As a result of these visits and my experience as a physician in the British National Health Service I have attempted to carry out what must be a very personal analysis and comparison of the three systems of medical care. The material has been collected from notes, from discussions and from reading – but in spite of the need for reliable comparisons there are few studies that have been carried out, for apart from the World Health Organisation there is no body encouraging such work, few local groups or organisations promoting meetings and discussions, few university departments engaged in this work and little support for such researches.

The contents deal with the general principles and philosophy of provision of medical care, with the components and the levels of administration and care. In all systems there are first-contact services providing primary care, specialist services for the ambulatory and hospitals. A section is devoted to each level and an analysis made of the ways in which the three systems provide these services. Two specific topics, maternity and child care and mental illness, are then taken to examine how care is provided in each system. The training and structure of the greater medical profession is described and finally some personal thoughts are given on future needs.

Each definitive chapter gives a general background of the topic, some questions that should be answered, the current state of services in the three systems, a comparison and some implications.

The difficulties of attempting to compare the three systems are recognised. Published statistics of health indices are known to be fallible and based on differing definitions, concepts and intentions. The observer-errors of a single observer who visited two foreign lands for the first and only time are recognised. Yet in spite of these possible deficiences and errors it is to be hoped that this book will serve a purpose in highlighting the need for more planned studies and researches into the field of comparative international medical care. If national prejudices can be overcome and co-

operation developed, then continuing operational studies
in depth and with sophistication should be developed.
Faced with common problems and dilemmas we shall make
the greatest progress by learning from one another.

John Fry
Beckenham. October 1969

Chapter 1
Medical Care

COMMON GOALS AND COMMON PROBLEMS

We live in a changing world that, with its social, technological, scientific and medical advances, is coming ever closer together in stating and defining its hopes and objectives.

In the developed societies of the world an educated and expectant public has emerged – expectant of a fuller life with all the benefits and comforts associated with modern living, and particularly high amongst these greater expectations is the desire to achieve and maintain health during a long and useful life. The charter of the World Health Organisation has stated that health, a state of physical, mental and social well-being, should be regarded as a human and civic right. Faced then with the challenge of providing this human right and meeting the expectations of their citizens, how have three of our greatest nations proceeded to tackle the problems? This is the essence of this book.

PROVISIONS OF MEDICAL CARE

Accepting that medical care and health maintenance are an important sector of public policy it is justifiable to approach the problems of description and comparison, first by stating some common hopes and difficulties, and then by analysing how three nations have tackled various aspects of medical care.

There is no one single health system that is best. Medical care is, just as any other social activity, closely related to local and national customs, beliefs and traditions. The health services of any nation have evolved over many generations as mirrors of national character. This must be accepted as an inevitable fact of modern life. Yet, even though the national characters of the USSR, USA and UK are different, there are many common factors by which their ways of providing care, and their achievements, can be compared.

Any observer of modern medical care systems visiting any country will soon discover that there exists a chorus of discontent.

In the USA there is considerable consumer dissatisfaction with the mounting costs of personal medical care that the ordinary man-in-the-street is excepted to meet. There is dissatisfaction with the quality of service received and there is evidence of poor relationships between the medical profession and the public.

In the UK, with its National Health Service (NHS), although there is apparently less consumer dissatisfaction than in the USA, there is greater dissatisfaction within the medical profession with the facilities available for modern medical care.

In the USSR the sound of discontent may be muted, but it is nevertheless, still evident to those who are able, and allowed, to listen. With some lessening of controls and constraints, dissatisfactions are beginning to be expressed over the lack of choice and selection in the medical services. From the medical profession are heard plaintive cries over the isolation of the Soviet doctors from their colleagues in the West, which is leading to difficulties and frustrations over the comparisons of techniques and methods of medical care.

In all countries dramatic scientific and technological advances outside medicine have had a particular impact on medical care, and there is general agreement particularly in these three nations that established and basic tenets must now be critically revaluated to see how best to meet the medical needs of a modern society.

COMMON GOALS – MAXIMUM HEALTH AT MINIMUM COST

The goal of all systems of medical care is to provide the highest possible quality of care commensurate with the least possible diversion of that society's resources from other goods and services.

Having stated this common endeavour there are immediate problems and difficulties.

What is meant by 'highest possible quality'? What proportion of available national resources should be used for care, cure or prevention of disease?

Even if agreement could be achieved on the common goals of medical care there is then the difficulty of measuring the extent to which these goals are met. Different answers, for example, will inevitably be obtained if consumer and professional satisfactions are measured.

Then there are difficulties related to the allocation of resources – not only in connection with economic factors, or the involvement of governments in planning medical services, but also in relation to the particular riches and resources of a country. Thus in the USA there is a comparative abundance of computers and other labour-saving devices which are being diverted and adapted to medical needs. In the USSR, on the other hand, there is a great wealth of relatively 'inexpensive' manpower, and even more woman-power, that has been recruited and directed to staff the medical care services. In the UK there are examples of the restrictive effects of historical traditions on a National Health Service that is new in concept but old in ideas and material facilities.

Then there are the difficulties associated with striking a balance between the minimum acceptable levels of quality and the maximum resources that can be allocated to medical care. It is evident that someone somewhere has to make decisions on priorities, and that somehow there have to be 'gatekeepers' restricting the rates of utilisation of services. Whether such decisions are made at the highest government levels or are left to less restrictive pricing mechanisms associated with private medical care will depend on a combination of the national political viewpoints and historical factors relative to that country.

It is evident, already, that faced with common goals and their associated problems, there must in any country be a strong incentive to make the best possible use of available resources.

Medical Care

The problems associated with common goals in medical care have been referred to – decisions on priorities of resources, the rising costs of services and consumer and professional dissatisfactions.

Yet no nation has so far resolved the modern doctors' dilemma of matching the '*wants*' of the consumers with the '*needs*' as defined by professional assessors and planners, with the '*resources*' that are available.

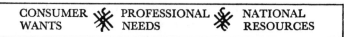

CONSUMER WANTS ✻ PROFESSIONAL NEEDS ✻ NATIONAL RESOURCES

Fig. 1. The insoluble equation of medical care.

The '*wants*' of consumers will depend not only on the obvious acute and chronic diseases that have to be managed but also on other factors unrelated to health or disease. The formulation of wants depends on traditional freedom of expression, on the educational development which enables various degrees of sophistication of care to be thought out and worked out, and on consumer priority decisions which have to balance other social wants, such as living comforts, holidays and age of retirement, with medical care.

In spite of the progress of modern technology and science in medicine, and in spite of the increased opportunities available for the care of the sick it is somewhat disarming to discover that ultimately what the sick person and his family seek from the medical care system and the criterion by which quality of care often is measured by the consumer, is kindly and personal care provided by physicians and nurses whom he knows and respects.

The health '*needs*' are those that are defined by professional researchers and planners based on studies of medical and social resources and utilisation.

Such calculations, when they are carried out, seek to provide acceptable norms and standards on which to base future planning.

Praiseworthy and necessary as these planning exercises

are, the whole subject of estimating future medical needs is riddled with fallacies and difficulties.

The first difficulty is that the needs prescribed are those by a professional scientist for others. They are those considered necessary for a mass population. They are those that have achieved their place in competition with other measurable social needs, such as housing, education, food, transport, full employment and leisure facilities. Imposition of priorities in terms of need is not always acceptable to individual members of the general public.

Then there is the dilemma of decision as to where to draw the line. Medical services represent a bottomless pit of expenditure. It is a fallacy to believe that the more money and resources that are put into medical services then a healthier population will result whose care will eventually cost less and less.

There exists a *'vacuum of sophistication'* in disease. Control of major disorders, such as infections, and social problems and poverty has not led to a utopian state of health and absence of disease. Into the vacuum created by control of tuberculosis and cancer, where this is possible, come crowding in a mass of other and increasingly sophisticated conditions such as emotional disorders, diseases of ageing and degeneration and social problems such a illegitimacy, crime and 'broken homes'.

There is a permanant *'mirage of health'* and it must be accepted that all systems of medical care will have to be planned to cope with insatiable needs and with built-in schemes for priority decisions.

The distribution of needs and utilisation of resources, have also been complicated by other factors such as the increasing professional trend towards specialisation which in turn has led to problems in providing primary medical care. Urbanisation is world-wide. More and more people are moving to live in large towns and the problems of caring for dispersed rural communities are increasing because of difficulties in attracting physicians into remote areas.

Ultimately the pattern and success of medical care rests on the ways in which the nationally available medical resources are deployed and utilised.

Faced with these common goals and problems how can

the medical services of the USSR, USA and UK be compared and contrasted?

Comparison of published national statistics relating to numbers and rates of hospital beds, physicians, nurses and other facilities only begins to show some of the differences between nations. Examination and analysis are necessary of the ways in which the systems are organised and administered and the services provided in order that something more meaningful may emerge.

These are two possible methods amongst others by which medical care can be compared. One endeavours to measure the outcome of care, that is its success as evident from common indices of health and social pathology. Comparisons can be made for example of such specific factors as infant mortality rates, of general mortality and morbidity and of the effects of various preventive schemes.

The advantage of such rates is that it represents the ultimate measures of effectiveness of medical care in any place.

Unfortunately there are a number of disadvantages to this method. Firstly rates are not strictly comparable. Their reliability depends on accurate definitions which are not common to all nations. Their reliability can be sound only where strictly comparable intensive prospective studies are carried out and this has not been possible yet on a wide scale.

Secondly, the 'outcomes' of medical care may not be equated with the actual care given. There are so many other uncontrolled factors, social and personal, as well as medical, that may influence the outcome that once again comparisons are difficult.

Thirdly, there are difficulties in deciding on the relevant measurements to be carried out. Apart from the common and rather crude indices there are others that are more refined and more difficult to measure. Thus, how is the final outcome of chronic illness to be measured – and what of consumer attitudes and satisfactions? If they are to be included in measuring outcome, how, and by what means are these inestimables assessed?

The other method of studying medical care is that of examining the *structure and functions* of the various national systems. Faced with certain problems of providing care, how do the services in the various nations tackle these common problems?

For example, how is first-contact care organised, or how are the services for the mentally sick carried out, or how is the challenge of prevention and early diagnosis being tackled?

The methods of comparison employed in this book are an inevitable compromise, for they are the report and findings of an individual professional observer. An observer who, as a practising British physician with a particular interest in medical care, was able to pay prolonged visits to the USA and USSR.

I have attempted to act as a recording machine to observe the countries and their national characters, to study the system and patterns of medical care organisation and administration, to examine the details of work at the various levels of care and to analyse the available data.

Each of the chapters seeks to consider the international background of the topic discussed followed by a factual description of the ways in which each of the three nations is tackling the problem. I then seek to make some comparisons between the three countries and finally to consider some of the implications of these comparisons.

Chapter 2
National Characteristics

Whilst standards of medical care are useful indices of social progress and advancement they must always be related to national characteristics and background.

Of particular influence on standards of medical care are geographical and population patterns: the historical evolution of national ideologies and traditional social, cultural and philosophical beliefs; the overall standards of living as they affect the daily lives of ordinary people; and the priorities given to different needs.

The USSR

The Union of Soviet Socialist Republics (USSR) is the world's largest nation. Covering an area of more than 8·6 million square miles it is two-and-a-half times the size of the USA. It extends from the ice-packed ports of Murmansk and Archangel in the north to the torrid deserts bording Iran and China in the south. From the modern European cities of Riga, Leningrad and Moscow on the west it extends through the forests and plains of Siberia to the Bering Straits in the east. The USSR possesses all known natural resources, with the exception of some tropical agricultural products. Its industries are spread and dispersed throughout the nation with half of its steel now coming from east of the Volga.

The 230 million Soviet citizens include a great variety of peoples of many backgrounds – slavonic, baltic, central asian and caucasian. Schoolchildren in the USSR are now being taught in no fewer than 61 different languages.

The vast land mass of the USSR, is relatively sparsely populated, with a population density of only 26 persons per square mile. About one-half of its population is said to be still 'rural' (46 per cent in 1966).

The USSR is an old nation with a new social and political system. Although its social history can be traced directly back more than 1,000 years to Koevan Russia, its modern history dates back only fifty years, to 1917.

The USSR is a federation of many old and ancient cultures and societies, each proud and sensitive of its own historical traditions. There is still no single Russia. The Georgians, the Ukrainians, the Armenians and the Uzbecs, whilst all Soviet citizens, also consider themselves as members of local societies.

Any assessment of progress and achievements must take note of the transition during fifty years and two world wars, from an inefficient autocratic agricultural serfdom to one of the world's leading technological nations.

However, an autocracy inherited from the Tartars and the Tsars is still to be found in the modern Soviet State. Thus the idolatry that surrounds Lenin – and his pictures and monuments are found in every corner of the USSR – has its origins in the adoration of the tsar, the 'little father'. The ideological base of political and social institutions may be new, but many of the practical forms that they take are buried deep within the cultures of past societies.

NATIONAL CHARACTERISTICS

An early impression that persists during a stay in the USSR, is that of a rich nation with poor people. There are ready and reasonable explanations.

In its fifty years, in order to achieve parity with the West, modern Russia has had to formulate and adhere to an agreed order of priorities according to the needs of the State. Consumer goods and comforts have inevitably occupied lower orders of importance then scientific, technological, agricultural, industrial and medical requirements.

These fifty years have been hard years. Whilst the actual 1917 revolution may have been relatively bloodless, the havoc and destruction of the Civil War that followed until 1923 and World War II, from 1941 to 1945, were disastrous.

It has been estimated that in the Civil War more than 10

million people were killed, or died of starvation or epidemics. In one account it was stated:

> "There were more than 20 million cases of typhus with 3 million deaths. In 1921 there were 200,000 cases of cholera, 300,000 of typhoid and more than 80,000 of smallpox. Syphilis assumed almost epidemic proportions. In 1922, in some sections of Russia, 80 per cent of the population were infected, and in 1923 in some districts of north western Russia, this percentage rose to 95 per cent. Scurvy also became rampant. . . . The total number of deaths from epidemics in Russia from 1916 to 1923 was between 8 and 10 million."

In World War II, most of what had been built up was destroyed again. More than 20 million Russians were killed on the battlefield or died through privation in occupied areas, a figure that represents more than 1 in 8 of the total population. As President John F. Kennedy noted in 1963:

> "No nation in the history of battle ever suffered more than the Soviet Union in the Scond World War. At least 20 millions lost their lives. Countless millions of homes of families were burned or sacked. A third of the nation's territory, including two-thirds of its industrial base was turned to wasteland, a loss equivalent to the destruction of the United States east of Chicago."

Yet, in twenty years all has been rebuilt and much more besides.

The effects of these struggles of the Russian peoples, not only those over the past fifty years but also the social miseries over centuries past, have to be appreciated and noted in describing and comparing current medical and other services.

Not only have these hardships created internal stresses but they have also influenced relationships with the outside world. A state of social isolation has developed with few exchanges between ordinary Russians and those in the Western nations. This isolation has had the effect of creating difficulties in self-appraisal and self-criticism. This applies particularly to the medical field in which much that is new is inextricably bound with much that is old and traditional.

There is much of both that has not yet been subjected to frank and critical analysis and evaluation.

BASIC PHILOSOPHIES

In the Soviet system the State is predominant and no competition with it is tolerated. A great monolithic organisation exists with national planning and executive policies.

Individuals and family life fit into a pattern of national priorities. Planning meets with few apparent difficulties or resentments by the majority of Soviet citizens.

The need for national priorities and personal restrictions and sacrifices has been accepted and great pride and confidence are felt now over achievements in Space travel and other modern endeavours.

Social isolation has inevitably created difficulties in relations with foreigners. There is suspicion and mistrust, but at the same time warm hospitality and pride in showing the achievements and successes of the past fifty years.

FAMILY LIFE AND PROBLEMS

For the Soviet citizen and his family there are similar basic problems, desires, dreams and aspirations of life as those facing Britons and Americans.

Survival and sustenance present few problems to the Russian. There are jobs for everyone who wants to work and officially there is no unemployment – only 'technological unemployment' with more sophisticated economic planning.

With overall employment there is a tendency for an underworked and often underpaid work-force. The average working day for the physicians as well as other workers is $6\frac{1}{2}$ hours and there is now a 5-day week.

Incomes in the USSR cannot be compared easily with those in the USA and UK since there is almost no income tax and much state subsidisation of housing, transport costs and, of course, free education and medical care. For example, rent of a town flat is only at a rate of 5–10 per cent of the worker's salary. Yet it is significant that though 'overtime' work is discouraged officially, 'after-hours', second, and even third jobs are customary, especially among the young, and, of course, many wives and mothers go out to work.

Families tend to be small. The birth rate in the USSR is falling and there is no 'population explosion'. In Moscow and Leningrad more than 2 children a family is unusual. The reasons are shortage of housing for larger families and because educated and trained women want to work.

Because young wives are encouraged to continue to work the grandmother becomes an important member of the family. She does the housework and some shopping. She is there when the children come home from school or during holidays. For the same reasons there is a very extensive network of State crèches, nursery schools and kindergartens where young children may be left during their mother's working hours.

Shortages of consumer goods and inefficiencies of the monolithic State retail organisation can make shopping a lengthy and frustrating daily experience. Queues have become an inevitable feature of life in modern Russia. Orderly queues are seen everywhere and much time and effort may be seen as being thus spent and wasted.

Compared with the West there are many fewer private motor cars, shops contain fewer quality products and window displays are unimaginative, uninspiring and unattractive. Advertisements and hoardings are conspicuous by their absence.

Cultural and sporting activities are however more popular than in the West, with many more opportunities for self-participation. Even the smallest towns have their own theatre and sports stadiums.

A great contrast between 'town' and 'country' still remains. Whilst life in urban USSR is not all that different from the cities of any other developed nation, rural Russia, where more than half of the population live, is still far behind the cities in social development.

The USA

The United States of America is currently the wealthiest nation on earth.

It is the fourth largest country in area (after the USSR, China and Brazil). Its 200 million Americans live in 3·6 million square miles and the population density of 55 per square mile is twice that of the USSR.

Stretching across the North American continent from the Atlantic to the Pacific Ocean and meeting Canada in the north and Mexico in the south, it has a climate ranging from temperate to semi-tropical.

The USA is a land full of wealth and resources. It vibrates with a sense of space and movement in which its 200 millions live, work and intermingle.

Although it has a relevant social history of three and a half centuries it is in fact a young nation because its main population growth occurred in the past one hundred years only.

A nation with tender and sensitive roots, it comprises peoples from many national backgrounds, customs and traditions. Few Americans can count more than one or two native-born generations in their ancestry. A mixture of British, Russian, Polish, Irish, Italian, Scandinavian, Spanish, German, African, Caribbean and Oriental origins, each of which contributes a significant proportion to the population, leads to much modern American life and political behaviour being orientated towards particular groups, none of which constitutes a clear majority of the population.

Although its two centuries of relative political stability, with only one major insurrection, the Civil War one hundred years ago, classifies it as an old nation amongst current governments, it is in most ways a very youthful and insecure society with an image of extrovertism, that is still feeling its way to a common national character. Its people are anxious about outside opinions, appreciative of praise, sensitive of comment and resentful of criticism.

BASIC PHILOSOPHIES

A prevalent legend is that which C. Van Woodward has called the "American legend of Success and Victory".

". . . Unique good fortune has isolated America, I think rather dangerously, from the common experience of the rest of mankind, all the great peoples of which have, without exception, known the bitter taste of defeat and humiliation.

It has fostered the tacit conviction that American ideals, values and principles inevitably prevail in the end . . . and this assumption exposes us to the temptation of believing that we are somehow immune from the forces of history."

The absence of a State religion or monarchy has led to considerable emphasis on 'loyalty'.

It is the very rare school-room that does not begin each day with a pledge of allegiance to the American flag. This constant repetition of allegiance to a flag, rather than to a person or to an ideological group or to a 'homeland', is a significant characteristic American social attitude.

Brought up on the sanctity of the Declaration of Independence and worship of the Stars and Stripes, it is scarcely surprising that free enterprise and individual freedom and liberty are dominant themes. With this goes emphasis on the responsibilities of the individual that must accompany freedom and liberty. Each American is expected to make a success of his life and to be able to provide for himself and his family when the needs arise. Success is synonymous with wealth.

Paradoxically, along with all the stress on loyalty and responsibility, there is great suspicion of 'government'. The Federal Government is despised by some just as local government is by others. In general the more conservative and authoritarian the group the greater the suspicion of Federal Government, and, the more liberal, integrationist and libertarian the group the greater the suspicion of State and local government.

SOCIAL PARADOX

The one universal criterion of success is visible wealth.

Yet, in the world's wealthiest society, with what other nations would consider almost a superfluity of resources, there is poverty, unemployment and misery perhaps greater in extent and degree than any now seen in other 'developed' countries.

The urgency of alleviating poverty, and in particular Negro poverty, has become evident in the recurrent riots since 1965. Although Negroes account for only 11 per cent of the population of the United States they suffer from a far higher proportion of social problems. With their illegitimacy rates of over 25 per cent of all live births, with less than one-half of Negroes at 18 living with their familes, with 20 per cent of Negro children 'fatherless' and with the community's highest rates of unemployment and illiteracy, legacies of years of neglect, it is not surprising to find personal, family and social instabilities with high crime rates.

Whilst much effort and activity have been apparent over the past few years in attempts to resolve these human problems, any success has been slow.

A block to many social programmes has been the great American emphasis that is placed on individual effort and achievement. In the free and democratic American society where there are, in theory, equal opportunities for all, it has been assumed rather naively by many success-ful Americans that failure or lack of success, as evident by the social problems and tangles that an individual suffers, are the results of deficiencies in his own personal character, rather than due to any defects in the structure of the Ameri-can way of life. Examples often are quoted of individuals who have 'lifted themselves' above their backgrounds, and, indeed, there are many instances of mobility within social class and geography. Yet, the great majority of those born to poverty are destined to remain poor, in opportunity as well as material goods throughout their lives.

There has been, until very recently, a public insensitivity over those social problems and circumstances considered to be within the individual's power to control. Conflicts of philosophies exist over matching individual actions and responsibilities, with public interference in the welfare of those less able to manage.

Hidden amongst the high level of total unemployment (up to 5–10 per cent of working age population in some areas) is partial employment, which is not recorded as 'unemploy-ment', and the general insecurity of the actual employment. Jobs appear much less secure in the United States than in the UK or the USSR. There exists a greater ruthlessness in American industry and commerce over the individual in relation to the company or corporation that employs him. There is a willingness to sacrifice individuals to the god of technical efficiency and material profits. New methods and new techniques can, and do, lead to unemployment of workers who may have given twenty or thirty years to the company and who at the age of 50 find new work difficult.

FAMILY LIFE AND PROBLEMS

The family is the basic social unit which in the United States is presided over by the Mother, who occupies a particularly prominent place of respect.

The ambitions of American family life are to remain in-dependent and solvent. The aims are to own their own home and eventually to pay for what they receive. The high levels of growing family needs do not match current incomes and much that is bought is done so on loans of various forms.

For those who are able to afford necessities the American way of life provides the highest level of consumer comfort in the world. High quality housing is expensive, there are more cars per population than anywhere else on earth, food is plentiful and there are good opportunities for leisure and travel. Education is free up to the university level. There is employment for skilled workers but with less long-term security. Americans are restless and in this highly mobile society it has been estimated that in some years up to 20 per cent of the population may be engaged in moving house from one town to another.

The United Kingdom

Compared with the two giants, the USSR and the USA, the United Kingdom is a tiny European off-shore island. It has an area of 90,000 square miles and its 54 million in-habitants create a population density of 575 per square mile – a density that is ten times that of the USA, and twenty-five times that of the USSR.

In spite of its small size the over-populated British Isles offer a special interest in comparison with the USSR and the USA.

The United Kingdom has had a longer social history than the USSR and the USA, and most of its present social and medical services have evolved out of many centuries of his-torical experience and endeavour.

The former ruler of an Empire, and now the mere titular

centre of the British Commonwealth, since its colonies have achieved independence, the United Kingdom is having to adjust to a new role in world affairs.

From relying on the wealth of colonial natural resources it now has to make its mark more as a trader, manufacturer, a commercial centre and a leader in technology, science and education.

A nation with many old customs and traditions, a birth-place of democracy and freedom, the UK faces the challenge of creating for itself a new place in the modern world.

As the leader in the Industrial Revolution and as the possessor of one of the first railway systems in the world, it now has to re-equip and readjust its railways to modern needs. As a leader in the development of hospitals over the past two centuries, it is faced now with the need to replace the old buildings with new.

The United Kingdom presents an example of an old society with sound and established traditions and customs that have been developed slowly over many centuries and that now have to be reshaped to new and modern needs and situations.

BASIC PHILOSOPHIES

Predominant in the British national character has been an emphasis on personal and individual freedom and rule by democracy through Parliament, with the monarchy occupying an increasingly less important role in the background.

Provision and supply of medical care and social aid have evolved and become adapted through changing sociological systems over the past 300 years. Changes from an agricultural society through the industrial revolution to the modern technological state have included changes in the medical and social services.

In the feudal and agricultural society it was the benevolent landlord or squire who was responsible, if he so wished, for arranging the simple medical services for his tenants and servants and it was he who made provisions to support his people in old age, infirmity and disability. The small and independent craftsmen and workers in the larger cities had to fend for themselves and make their own arrangements.

With the industrial revolution of the eighteenth and nineteenth centuries, the shift from the rural to urban and industrial life created major problems of medical and social care. It was in the grimy industrial cities that medical insurance schemes were born, with the 'sick clubs' organised by well-meaning employers or trade groups and unions. For a few pence each week as capitation fees local doctors thus undertook to provide basic care for workers and their families.

In 1911 this philosophy was accepted by the State through the National Health Insurance Act, which ensured medical care for all workers below a certain level of income. Under this Act those workers could 'register' with a general practitioner who undertook to provide general medical care for an annual capitation fee. The workers' families were not included in this scheme.

Finally, in 1948 the last phase of this evolutionary process occurred with the introduction of the National Health Service (NHS) as part of the Welfare State. Under the NHS all medical care was to be provided free at time of need. The whole population could receive general medical care from general practitioners, with whom they would register and for whose care the physician would receive an annual capitation fee. The hospitals became a single national co-ordinated service.

With the NHS there was a great expansion of other associated social and welfare services, such as the development of social agencies, better unemployment and disability assistance, provisions for better care in old age and services for children, provision for better housing and education.

The Welfare State is now twenty-one years old and all teenagers are now the products of this system. It has become an immovable part of the modern British way of life. Politicians may tinker with it but it is past the stage of abolition or replacement by an alternative system based on free enterprise and individual responsibilities.

FAMILY LIFE AND PROBLEMS

The family is accepted as the fundamental social unit. This is acknowledged by the State through family allowances, special tax and other concessions.

Following a post-World War II boom the birth rate has

now fallen and the average family now comprises 2 or 3 children.

Family life has been markedly influenced by the Welfare State but individual freedom of action remains. Although education is free, there is much housing provided by local government and medical care is free and readily accessible under the NHS – there still exist thriving private schools, more than one-half of the population live in owner-occupied homes and it is estimated that up to 5 per cent of the population choose to arrange for private medical care outside the NHS.

Yet, in spite of the altruistic dreams of the Welfare State there still exist many social problems and frustrations. These may nevertheless be more related to the present difficulties of the readjustment of the United Kingdom in its new role in the world than to any special shortcomings of the principle of the Welfare State.

Comparisons

For summary then it may be said that the USSR is a totalitarian society with the State as the overall controller and planner, and because of this there is limitation of freedom with economic and political power in a few hands. There is a noteworthy absence of competition in all major fields of endeavour. Progress and planning are based on the application of agreed national priorities which are decided upon at the highest hierarchical levels.

Its achievements over fifty years have been enormous, for from an old and backward serf-like Tsarist autocracy it has become one of our leading technological and scientific nations.

The USA by contrast is a young nation still searching for its soul. Although it is the world's wealthiest nation it still has great social prolems and is only slowly beginning to resolve them.

A national philosophy, based on free enterprise and individual liberty with responsibility, has allowed a policy of laissez-faire to develop which has been reasonably satisfactory to those who have been successful, but very hard on those who have failed.

National Characteristics

The UK is an old nation with a society built on traditions and customs of the past. It is faced with difficulties in readjusting its changed international and economic position to meet the modern needs of the country. It has sought to meet its social needs through a Welfare system that offers full medical and social services to all its people.

Chapter 3
Structure and Patterns of Medical Services

To live a full life that is both enjoyable to the individual and useful to the community in a modern society men and women now expect a system of medical care, on which they may call in time of need that is interested and concerned in preventing disease, and that provides all the necessary services for their social and welfare requirements.

Medical care is expensive, and now much of it is quite out of reach of the ordinary pocket. No family now can afford to pay for anything more than a small fraction of the total cost of a moderate, let alone a major, illness. The cost of one week's stay in a modern hospital is two or three times that of the weekly income of an average family.

For this reason, and because it is necessary to make the best use of available services through planning, there must be increasing government involvement in the provision of medical services for any community.

It is however impossible, even with government funds, to provide all the medical wants and needs of everyone. Somehow and somewhere brakes have to be applied and reasonable priorities accepted.

Faced with these common situations how have our three nations, the USSR, the USA and the UK proceded to meet the problems? What common denominators exist and what lessons can we learn from one another?

THE BASIC PRINCIPLES AND COMPONENTS OF ANY
'HEALTH SERVICE'

It is necessary first to clarify the fundamental principles

that underlie the provision of medical care. These will be influenced by national attitudes but it is necessary, for any comparison, to know how the services are paid for and how they are planned in order that they may be available and accessible to all.

All medical services can be divided into a series of levels of care, depending on the specialist expertise required and the following levels may be recognised:

(i) *The Family*

It is within the family that the first steps are taken towards medical care, prevention of disease and health maintenance. National attitudes vary and so do the policies taken to support and encourage the family as a strong unit.

Under current discussion internationally is the importance, for example, that is placed on providing continuing care for the family as a single unit by a single health team.

(ii) *Doctor-of-First-Contact*

In all systems of medical care some medically qualified person has to provide the first professional contact with the patient. These doctors-of-first-contact encounter a spectrum of morbidity that is quite different from that seen at more specialised and hospital levels. At this first-contact level patients present with vague and unstructured symptoms often unrelated to any special categories of disease. The majority of the illnesses occurring at this level are relatively minor and do not require any real specialised care.

Working in a relatively small and static population, compared with that of a hospital, these doctors will obviously be concerned more with the common diseases of man than esoteric rarities. They will tend to provide long-term and continuing care for their patients, in contradistinction to the short-term and transient care provided at hospitals.

(iii) *Specialist Services for the Ambulatory (Out-patient Services)*

The next level of care is the specialist who restricts his work more to specific diseases, or age and sex groups of the population. As a rule the specialist provides care for a much larger segment of the population than does the doctor-of-first-contact, since the more specific disorders for which specialist care is required are less frequent, because they have been pre-selected.

(iv) *Hospitals*

The hospitals are the modern centres for the most complex and most expensive forms of medical care. Traditionally acting as shelters for the sick poor they now have many other functions, such as local centres for diagnostic procedures, and the professional research and education of the medical under- and post-graduate.

(v) *Community and Public Health Medical and Social Services*

In general these have a supporting role for the traditional clinical patterns of medical care, but their role is altering as medical care becomes more sophisticated.

The Structure of the Health Service in the USSR

Health Services were given an important priority in planning new social policies in the USSR in 1917.

The principles on which medical care has been developed are as follows:

1. Medical Care is planned and developed on socialist and economic philosophies. As an integral part of the national socio-economic programme medical care takes its place amongst all the other plans and developments on which the socialist Soviet State is run.

2. Medical Care is '*free*' to all at the time of need, although some nominal payments are required for drugs, dentures, spectacles and certain surgical appliances – but almost one-half of the population are exempt from these charges, i.e. children, invalids and war veterans.

3. Medical Care is available and accessible to all. This probably has been the greatest achievement of the Soviet medical system. To ensure that care is available and accessible to all the 230 million Soviet citizens even in the remote rural areas has required major planning, deployment and direction of resources.

4. Medical Care is carried out by '*specialists*' who are well qualified, and who have undergone a lengthy professional training – in the case of physicians the training is six

c

years. Specialisation down to the first-contact level was accepted as a principle in the late 1930s and the whole medical system has been based on this concept, commencing with special education for medical students. Students have to select one of three specialist faculties – general medicine, paediatrics or public health – in which to carry out their medical studies from the time that they enter medical school at 18–19 years of age.

5. Great emphasis is placed on *prevention* in all fields of medical care. Unity of preventive and curative services is the goal. This principle of prevention extends right through the whole system involving physicians in hospitals and industry as well as doctors-of-first-contact.

The chief techniques of disease-prevention and health promotion include – preventive immunisation and environmental control; regular screening of individuals in vulnerable groups; an extension of the screening programme in which certain groups of the population are followed up carefully over many years (see Chapter 7); and health education, using modern media such as television, puppet theatres and posters, with physicians being expected to devote up to an hour of each working day in this work.

6. The aim of health education is to create a co-operative public, knowledgeable in the basic elements of health maintenance and disease prevention. It is also intended to achieve *active involvement and participation of the public* in medical care, in such exercises as the maintenance of standards of hygiene and sanitation, ensuring follow-up attendances at clinics and the application and enforcement of public health policies. Such activities are carried out by health volunteers who also give their time to work in hospitals and polyclinics.

BASIC STRUCTURE

The aims of the Soviet system of medical care are to meet these stated principles and to ensure that modern health services are available to all citizens.

In order to achieve these objectives medical services have been tightly organised into discrete administrative levels. These levels of care comprise first-contact care; specialist care for the ambulatory; and hospital services. The intentions are to achieve close integration and inter-relationships between the various parts of the system.

To ensure universal availability and accessibility an important concept is the peripheral territorial and neighbourhood area – the 'UCHASTOK'. This is the smallest unit of care and there are some 60,000 such *uchastoks* in the USSR, 1 to every 4,000 persons, all served with medical services. This territorial *uchastok* principle also extends to industrial units, which, if large enough, organise their own medical services which are sited at the industrial centre.

In order to understand the Soviet system a description of the *flow of care* through the various levels is necessary. (Fig. 2.)

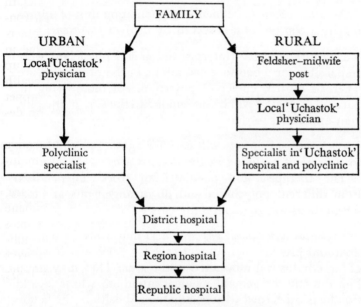

Fig. 2. Flow of medical care in the USSR.

1. *The Family*

The intention of widespread health education is to inculcate considerable self-help in the individual and his family. This applies more to health maintenance and disease prevention than to self-treatment of established disease.

There is no evidence in the USSR of attempts to discour-

25

age, limit or restrict the use of available medical services. The Soviet people are encouraged to seek medical advice when they consider it necessary and home visiting is considered a necessary and important part of care. (This has led to a very high rate of utilisation of first-contact services. (Chapter 4.))

The 'family' is not considered as a single unit requiring a single and distinct 'family doctor' and it has access to a number of possible first-contact physicians.

2. *First-Contact Services*

First-contact care is based on the *uchastok* (neighbourhood area) principle.

An *urban uchastok*, defined as a population unit of approximately 4,000 persons, is served by its own *physicians*:

– a *uchastok therapist* (internist or general physician) who is responsible for 2,000 to 2,500 adults in the prescribed area. There is no free choice of physician. All those living in a particular *uchastok* will be designated to the care of the physician appointed to that area.

– a *uchastok paediatrician* will care for 750–1,250 children up to the age of 15 living in the defined area.

The therapist and paediatrician work independently from different polyclinics and no arrangements are made for contacts to provide 'family care'.

– a *uchastok occupational physician* also may work in the same area and provide first-contact care for 1,000–2,000 workers of large industrial units sited in the area. They may consult him directly for general medical attention, whilst in addition he is concerned with occupational health in the factory.

The Urban *uchastok* physicians work from local polyclinics. They have special rooms and equipment provided there and each physician has a nurse working with him who assists in the clerical as well as the professional work.

In large cities such as Moscow, Leningrad and Kiev there are separate polyclinics for children and adults and others for psychiatric disorders, for skin and venereal diseases, for obstetric and gynaecological conditions, for tuberculosis and for neoplasms. There is thus considerable splintering of first-contact care. Patients may proceed directly to these specialist polyclinics (or dispensaries) without referral by their *uchastok* physician.

There is no sign or trend of any family teams providing co-operative care for the family group as a whole and it is not considered necessary to reintroduce any family physician.

In rural areas the difficulties of providing care for widely scattered populations make it impossible for the physician to act as the regular first medical contact. A system of para-medical auxiliary care has been built up. In all rural areas there are feldsher–midwife *posts* staffed by personnel classified as middle-grade medical staff with nursing and medical training, and a midwife responsible for antenatal and post-natal care and supervision of infants. (See Chapter 4.)

The feldsher–midwife posts are in close communication with, and under the supervision of, *uchastok* physicians, based on the local polyclinic or hospital.

3. *Specialist Care for Ambulatory Patients* is provided at the polyclinics. Working in the same building as the *uchastok* physicians are specialists such a surgeons, ophthalmologists, psychiatrists, oto-rhino-laryngologists and others, to whom patients may be referred or to whom patients may proceed in the first instance.

These specialists, except in rural areas, work only in the polyclinics and have no regular hospital duties or access to hospital beds. In rural areas where the polyclinic is combined with a small local (or *uchastok*) hospital there is a common medical staff for the combined unit.

The polyclinic is the medical centre in the community. It provides both first-contact and specialist services in the same building.

4. *Hospitals*

Hospitals in the USSR are primarily concerned with in-patient care. Out-patient services for ambulatory patients are at polyclinics that combine first-contact and specialist care. One local polyclinic is often built within the grounds of a *District* (*rayon*) hospital, but even here the two are distinct with different staffs and separate organisations for the polyclinic and the hospital.

The need for integration is recognised and the *Chief Physician of the District (rayon) hospital* is responsible for the organisation and administration of the whole of the local medical care services, including polyclinics, public health services and hospitals.

Soviet hospitals are graded according to the degrees of care that they are able to provide.

In rural areas there are many small Local (*uchastok*) hospitals, with from 10 to 100 beds. They are combined with polyclinic services and linked to feldsher–midwife posts.

In all areas the first-level large hospitals, with from 300 to 1,250 beds, are the *District (rayon)* hospitals. These are general hospitals with full facilities to deal with common acute and non-acute medical surgical, gynaecological and obstetric conditions.

More specialised hospital units such as thoracic surgery, cardiology and neurology and neurosurgery are sited at *Regional (oblast)* hospitals. Patients are normally referred to these *Regional* hospitals only through *District* hospitals, direct admissions are exceptional.

At the pinnacle of hospital hierarchy are the *Republic* hospitals which serve as the teaching hospitals and medical schools (institutes) in each of the fifteen Soviet republics. There may be more than one such hospital in any administrative or geographical republic, depending on its size.

PUBLIC HEALTH SERVICES

In addition to first-contact, specialist services, and hospitals, there are in all areas public health services organised through the *Sanepid (sanitary and epidemiological) system* (see Chapters 7 and 8), and occupational and industrial health services organised through special *medical-sanitation units* sited at larger industrial establishments.

These public health units are integrated with the clinical services and are administered locally with the hospital and the first-contact services by the Chief Physician of the District.

ADMINISTRATION OF HEALTH SERVICES

The administration and organisation of the Soviet health services correspond exactly to the general structure of central and local government, because they are integral parts of central and local government services.

Based on a hierarchical system of size, area, and diminishing responsibilities it is very much like the traditional Russian wooden doll, where wooden dolls of the same shape but diminishing size fit into one another. So it is with the Soviet health services. Starting with the Ministry of Health and extending down to the most peripheral and smallest units the pattern is similar in shape and form.

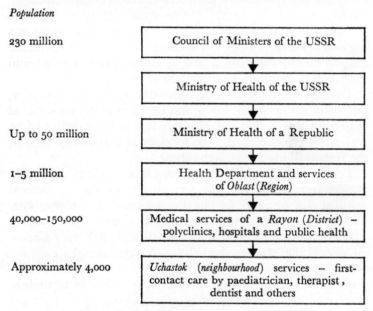

Population

230 million	Council of Ministers of the USSR
	Ministry of Health of the USSR
Up to 50 million	Ministry of Health of a Republic
1–5 million	Health Department and services of *Oblast (Region)*
40,000–150,000	Medical services of a *Rayon (District)* – polyclinics, hospitals and public health
Approximately 4,000	*Uchastok (neighbourhood)* services – first-contact care by paediatrician, therapist, dentist and others

Fig. 3. Structure of medical services in the USSR.

1. *Council of Ministers of the USSR*

At the highest level the central administrative unit is the Council of Ministers of the Union of Soviet Socialist Republics (USSR) and the Minister of Health is a member of the Praesidium or Cabinet.

2. *The Ministry of Health*

The Ministry of Health of the USSR has its headquarters in Moscow and is under the direction of the Minister of Health.

The Minister has always been an eminent practising doctor and the present holder is a thoracic surgeon with an international reputation, who still, whilst holding office, continues to operate and to teach. There are six Deputy Ministers of Health with departmental responsibilities.

The role of the USSR Ministry of Health is long-term planning and policy decisions on health services for 230 million Soviet citizens. Included in such decisions are the calculations and publication of norms and standards for resources and qualitative standards of medical care throughout the country.

The Ministry is responsible for the nation's health budgeting and defining priorities in keeping with national economic growth and development, and it collaborates closely with the Central Planning Council (GOSPLAN).

The staff of 900, of which two-thirds are physicians, is proportionately small for a nation of 230 millions. The reason for this is that the Ministry is a policy-making body and one not concerned with local administration which is the responsibility of the Republics.

The Ministry of Health is involved in medical education and is responsible directly for 10, out of the 85, Soviet medical schools and for 13 Postgraduate Institutes. The others are under the authority of local Republics.

A large Standing Medical and Scientific Advisory Council advises the Minister and the more professional Academy of Medical Services of the USSR on which the most eminent physicians serve as invited members, is available to undertake research studies and projects.

3. *Ministry of Health of Soviet Republics*

The USSR is divided into 15 republics. Each republic has its own Ministry of Health headed by a Minister who is appointed by the Central Soviet of the Republic, subject to the approval of the Minister of Health of the USSR.

The republics vary greatly in size and in population and in the nature of their geographical and medical problems. They extend from those in Western Europe to others in the Far East and the Arctic.

The budgets of each individual republic are derived from central government funds and are not based on any local taxation. The State is the sole trading agency and the owner of all natural riches. Taxation plays a small part in the financing of community and health services in the USSR.

4. *Regional (oblast) Health Department*

Detailed administration is carried out at regional levels, where the administrative unit is the *oblast*. The size of a Region ranges from 1 to 5 million persons. Large cities such as Leningrad, with a population of nearly 4 million, function as *oblasts*.

The Region has an Executive Council of members elected by the population. The Chief Medical Officer of the Region is an elected member of the Executive Council, and it is a full-time administrative appointment with responsibility for all the health services and institutions of the Regions – these include all polyclinics and dispensaries, hospitals and sanepids (public health services).

Responsibility for the various clinical specialist services in the whole *oblast* is allocated to the chiefs of the clinical departments at the main Regional hospital. For example, the Director of Surgery is responsible for the organisation and quality of surgical work in the Region. He maintains contact with and supervision of all surgeons and is responsible for ensuring adequate postgraduate training. In the same way the chiefs of the other departments are responsible for their specialist services within the Region.

5. *District (rayon) Health Services*

The Region is too large a unit for effectual day-to-day management of the various health services and is divided into districts serving populations of 40,000 to 150,000, which thus represent the basic peripheral administrative unit.

The District may have a single central hospital, but often there are several hospital units, a number of polyclinics and at least one public health unit.

All these health facilities are under the direction of the Chief Physician of the District. As a rule he is the senior physician of the central District hospital but he may be appointed from the polyclinic or public health services, and is directly responsible to the Chief Medical Officer of the Region.

6. Local (Uchastok) Care

The whole system of medical care rests on the concept of *uchastok* neighbourhood areas where personal care of the people is the responsibility of small teams or groups of medical and paramedical workers.

BUDGETING

Budgeting is an annual exercise that begins in the Districts where the Chief Physician, assisted by lay administrators, prepares a statement of his estimated needs and expenses according to national norms and standards, supplied by the Ministry of Health of the USSR. This statement is then passed on to the Region's health committee for approval, and at this level the budgets of all the Districts in the region are checked, correlated and adjusted. These estimates are then submitted to the Ministry of Health of the Republic for approval and further additional adjustments to meet special local needs. Finally, each Soviet Republic submits its budgets and estimates to the Ministry of Health of the USSR for final agreement.

Since the estimates and plans are all based on norms and standards produced by the Ministry it is unusual for much time to be spent on discussing cuts. On the contrary more often additions are made for extra services considered necessary by authorities at the higher levels.

The national accounting of the USSR is not based on gross national products but it is reported that of the total annual budget in 1966, 7·1 per cent was devoted to 'health and physical culture'.

PLANNING

Prospective planning of the health services of the USSR has been based on attempts to calculate the health needs of the people, through a variety of operational and statistical techniques.

Definition of needs has been based on a series of norms, standards and quotas. (For details see G.A. Popov in *The*

Efficiency of Medical Care, World Health Organisation, Regional Office for Europe, EURO, *294*, 2, 1967.)

Armed with such indices each area determines its deficiencies in relation to such indices and makes plans to meet them.

In practice, the planning of medical services in the USSR is a total operation combining central guidance with local action.

In each District a '*health inventory*' is carried out every five years when the standards of equipment, staffing, premises and various social facilities are measured and recorded. This exercise is carried out by the local 'public health' services under the direction of the Chief Physician of the District. Deficiencies are estimated and planning for the next five years is based on attempts to attain national standards and norms.

Similar exercises are carried out at the higher Regional and Republic levels and eventually a national plan is established and agreed. Once approved requirements are translated into needs of recruitment, educational facilities, and institutions such as polyclinics and hospitals, with final implementation carried out in each Republic under the general guidance of the Ministry of Health of the USSR.

Planning, therefore, involves all levels in the health services; it is based on assessments of needs and attempts to meet these; and any actions can be taken in the immediate and not in the far-distant future.

QUALITY CONTROLS

Control of quality of medical care in the USSR has been attempted through the definition of needs and the ways that they are met through the objective indices of national standards, norms and quotas. In addition, consumers' subjective feelings and opinions are safeguarded through public representation on governing committees at all levels.

ACCESSIBILITY AND CHOICE

In the Soviet medical system a compromise has been necessary between the provision of accessible services to all and the free choice of doctor. Free choice has been sacrificed so that a planned service available to all can be provided.

The medical profession in the USSR has less independence than in the USA and UK.

Physicians are considered as an expert professional and technical group of workers with defined and agreed tasks to perform like other professional and technical groups such as teachers, engineers and scientists. There are no special privileges for medical staff.

The medical profession has a trade union representation and organisation that safeguards and protects the individual physician and the professional group as a whole.

The status of the medical profession is high in the eyes of the public and there is a great demand for places in the medical schools. There are said to be 5–6 applicants for each place in medical schools in the USSR.

RESOURCES

The current (1966/67) stated medical resources in the USSR are shown in Table 1.

TABLE 1

Medical resources in the USSR

Population	230 million
Physicians	550,000 24 per 10,000 population
Annual number of new medical graduates	30,000 12 per 100,000 population
Nurses	35 per 10,000 population
Paramedical workers	37 per 10,000 population
Hospital beds	9·6 per 1,000 population

The Structure of the Health Services in the USA

Medical services in the USA until recently, have been allowed to evolve and develop according to local abilities and desires to meet local needs – as determined by local citizens.

It is only since 1966 that, with the enactment of Medicare and Medicaid legislation, there has been any widespread and significant government involvement in the provision of medical care and service. In the USA, by contrast with the USSR, there is no single system or pattern of care but a plurality of systems.

PRINCIPLES

1. Medical care provisions fit into the national concepts of free enterprise and free choice coupled with individual responsibilities. It has been left, wherever possible, to the individual to make his own arrangements for providing his own medical care and paying for it.

2. Traditional suspicions of, and antagonism towards the 'government' and the 'state', by the public and by the medical profession have prevented the Federal authorities from involvement in any planned and co-ordinated national system of medical care.

3. Planning of health services has been a compromise between laissez-faire policies associated with free enterprise and self-help national planning to ensure optimal utilisation with the assistance from central funds to meet the rising costs of medical care.

4. Payment for medical services has been on a 'fee-for-service' basis. The individual is given the ultimate responsibility, unless he is poor and classed as a 'medical indigent'. There are many variants. Many Americans now subscribe voluntarily to insurance schemes. There are voluntary group schemes involving occupational and other sections of the population and now there are government Medicare and Medicaid services to assist the elderly and the poor.

5. Accessibility and availability of services depend on local factors. They depend on the ability of small communities to attract physicians to settle. They depend on local wealth and the initiative and drive to provide local hospitals and medical centres. They depend on local geography and social factors.

6. Specialisation is the current fashion in the American

35

medical profession. Care is provided by highly trained 'specialists' from the first contact level upwards.

7. Attempts are made to ensure *quality and standards* of medical care through a range of procedures evolved gradually to safeguard at the same time as the patient, the providers of finance, the insurance companies and the federal authorities.

8. In addition to recognised public health procedures, *preventive care* involves regular 'medical check-ups' for those groups of the population able to meet the costs of such services or for those covered by special schemes that are part of their employment, or else included in a pre-paid insurance scheme.

9. Self-help and public involvement in medical care are encouraged as praiseworthy social endeavours but there is no overall organisation.

BASIC STRUCTURE

The structure in the American medical services appears untidy and confusing at first glance. All the necessary and recognised ingredients are there – hospitals, public health services, first-contact physicians and other units of social and paramedical care – but they are connected loosely in rather informal and unstructured ways that depend very much on local customs, beliefs and resources.

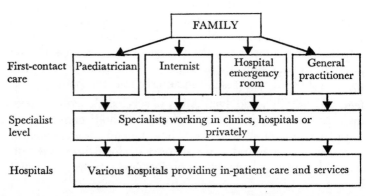

Fig. 4. Flow of medical care in the USA.

There is no uniform and overall structure of medical services in the USA. (Fig. 4 depicts the current situation.)

1. *The Family*

The family is recognised as an important and basic social unit and national policies are related to the integrity and support of the intra-family ties. Paradoxically, whilst emphasis is placed on the importance of the family as a single social unit this concept of 'unity' is not carried into the field of medical care.

The overall generalist and wide-ranging 'family doctor' has been replaced by a coterie of 'specialoids' each caring for different members of the family. The family is responsible for arranging its own medical care in a free market unless it is poor and recognised as medically indigent, when subsidised services are available.

2. *First-Contact Services*

First-contact care is of various types that depend on locality, wealth and customs.

In urban areas it is customary for children to be cared for by a paediatrician, parents by an internist, mother by an obstetrician-gynaecologist and all the family by various other specialists such as dermatologists, psychiatrists, ophthalmologists and oto-rhino-laryngologists who may be consulted directly by the family.

These physicians are selected freely and independently by the family and their services are paid for by fees-for-services that are the patients' responsibility.

For those who are unable to meet the costs of private personal services there are emergency rooms in the larger local hospitals which offer either free services or, for nominal fees, service from the staff in such departments, that is made up largely of trainee physicians.

In rural areas or in small urban communities there are fewer physicians and services available and there is little, if any, choice for the patient. In such circumstances there may be a single physician who acts as a generalist to provide 'family care' for all his patients.

37

3. *Specialist Care for Ambulatory Patients* is available readily in the cities.

Recognised specialists, with recognised specialist board certificates, may be consulted directly by the patients, or patients may be referred to them from other physicians.

Such specialists may work independently from private premises, in a group, in a large clinic or from a hospital.

As a general rule specialists have access to local hospitals where they may treat their patients.

4. *Hospitals*

There is a great range of hospitals in the USA from very large and special institutions, such as one mental hospital of 11,000 beds, to small local rural hospitals of 5–10 beds.

Some are administered by the State, some depend on voluntary contributions and others are organised as private profit-making establishments. The chief services are connected with in-patient care. A feature of American hospitals is that their services are available directly to most local physicians. There is no clear definitive separation of physicians in the USA into 'hospital' and 'non-hospital' doctors. This enables continuity of care to be provided by the physician.

The relations of a hospital with the local community depend on the locality. In many places the hospital is, at the same time, the medical centre supported and administered by local citizens.

ADMINISTRATION AND ORGANISATION

The administrative levels of medical care in the USA relate to national, geographical and population divisions.

At the highest level are the Federal agencies followed by State, City and more local services. However, although these levels can be defined, their inter-relations are variable and often tenuous and there is no recognisable and universal structure that can be applied to the whole nation.

1. *National Federal Agencies*

The central national government unit for medical care is the Department of Health, Education and Welfare (HEW). There is no separate Ministry of Health.

The public health division of this Department is headed by the Surgeon-General who, in turn, is responsible to the Secretary, who is a member of the government.

The Surgeon-General is a full-time civil servant and a physician with considerable public health experience.

The functions of the HEW public health division are limited strictly by design. They concern the giving of advice and information to other medical care organisations; the division supports and carries out considerable research work on scientific, clinical and operational subjects, not only in the USA but also abroad; and it finances certain specific and defined medical care projects that fit national policies.

Until the advent of Medicare and Medicaid the Federal agencies had little power or opportunity to undertake planning and organisation of total care services. The Bureau of Medical Services of the Department was involved chiefly in co-ordinating services between the separate States. Since 1946 however, the Division of Hospital Facilities has been able to influence the planning and development of hospitals through the Hill-Burton Act, under which hospital building in under-populated areas could be supported by Federal Funds.

2. *State Services*

Each of the fifty United States has its own self-governing public health services.

Each State Department of Health and Public Welfare is concerned with safeguarding the public's health through accepted sanitary and health measures and is responsible for making available certain basic medical services for indigents, and with implementing Medicare and Medicaid.

Under Medicare, the elderly are able to have a proportion of hospital costs and of personal medical services reimbursed from public funds.

The Medicaid system is intended to offer funds to those classified as needy 'medical indigents' to meet hospital and personal medical costs.

State public health departments are concerned also in the control of infectious diseases and in the care and supervision of mental illness, through preventive measures and by pro-

D

vision of State mental hospitals. Local nursing, maternity and child welfare services are also provided for those who seek them, namely, those who are not able to make private arrangements for such services.

3. *Regional and District Services*

More peripherally, health services are provided by cities, municipalities and counties. These divisions cover populations varying from a few thousand in rural areas to millions in the case of large cities such as New York, Chicago and Los Angeles.

The services provided by such regional and district authorities are similar, though on a smaller scale, to those provided by the states.

4. *Local (neighbourhood) Services*

Services at this level depend entirely on social factors such as the ability to pay for private medical care and on the availability of organised services for certain groups such as veterans, workers belonging to unions such as the Teamsters, and indigents.

BUDGETING

Payment for medical care in the USA comes from a variety and multiplicity of sources. There are private and public sectors. Private expenditure accounts for the largest share (74 per cent of total expenditure). In addition to these two clear-cut divisions there are various special pre-paid insurance schemes such as those organised by trade unions and other occupational groups for their members; health services organised by universities for their pupils, staff and families, and the veterans organisation, a federal service for ex-servicemen and their families.

TABLE 2

Expenditure for health and medical care as percentage of gross national product (GNP)

	1950	1955	1960	1965
Percentage of GNP	4·6	4·7	5·4	5·9

(Source: US Bureau of the Census, *U.S.A. 1967*.)

Expenditure on health and medical care has risen proportionately every year since 1950 (Table 2), and in 1965 it accounted for 5·9 per cent of the gross national product. With the new Medicare and Medicaid services it is now (1969) well over 6 per cent.

The proportions of the total annual expenditure of $38·5 billion accounted for by various sectors of the health service are shown in Table 3.

TABLE 3

Percentages of US health expenditure by object (1964)

Hospitals	35 per cent
	(Federal, 4 per cent;
	State, 11 per cent;
	Non-government, 20 per cent)
Physicians' services	20 per cent
Dental services	6 per cent
Drugs	12 per cent
Spectacles and appliances	3 per cent
Nursing homes	3 per cent
Medical research	4 per cent
Others	17 per cent

(Source: US Bureau of the Census, *U.S.A. 1967.*)

Out of the total private consumer expenditure on medical care (74 per cent of all costs for health and medical care in the USA) only one-third was covered by pre-paid insurance benefits. This proportion of insurance cover has risen from 12 per cent in 1950, through 27 per cent in 1960, to 33 per cent in 1964.

Most insurance benefits are for hospital care services (Table 4).

TABLE 4

Proportions of costs for hospital care and physicians' services in the USA (1964) met by insurance

	Direct payments	Insurance benefits
Hospital care	31 per cent	69 per cent
Physicians' services	62 per cent	38 per cent

(Source: US Bureau of the Census, *U.S.A. 1967.*)

In summary, the bulk of the expenditure on medical care in the USA is still met by the private consumer. Only one-third of these private consumer costs are covered by pre-paid insurance and that is chiefly for hospital care.

PLANNING

As noted, there have been few opportunities for overall planning of medical services.

At the national level planning is really at an interim phase. With the introduction of Medicare and Medicaid there may be new possibilities of influencing planning in the future through the Government's financial resources, but, until now, apart from the Hill-Burton Act of 1946 allowing some direction over planning of hospitals in under-developed areas, the Department of Health has been powerless to plan, and without any power to direct any groups or organisations.

At the *State* level it is only in the public health field that any planning has been possible and this has been patchy and local. More recently since the new legislation planning of services for medical indigents has started.

Locally, planning has depended on local leadership, initiatives, affluence and politics rather than on any desires to make best use of available resources.

There are some special examples by a few groups to plan medical services for their consumers.

In New York the *Health Insurance Plan* (HIP) provides pre-paid insurance medical care for nearly 750,000 persons. This it does through a series of group medical centres for first-contact and specialist ambulant services and through contracts and arrangements with local hospitals for hospital care.

In California the *Kaiser Permanente Scheme* provides similar services on a voluntary insurance basis.

In Detroit the *Community Health Association*, in co-opera-tion with trade unions of the motor workers, provides its own ambulatory and hospital services. There are in addition many voluntary medical groups and clinics, trade union schemes and the services for veterans provided by Federal authorities in which planning of care is evident, but they cover a small proportion of the population and there is no real link-up or co-operation between the various groups.

QUALITY CHECKS

A special feature of medical care in the USA is the large number of various built-in checks of quality of care.

Examinations and assessments by various specialist boards control the training and quality of specialists.

Prescribed standards for accreditation of hospitals serve as criteria for recognition for postgraduate training of physicians and for acceptance by insurance organisations.

Surgical work is checked by tissue committees that examine specimens removed at surgical operations, to check on the accuracy of diagnosis and on the criteria employed for undertaking surgical procedures.

Medico-legal claims occur at a higher rate than in the UK and the professional insurance premiums paid by physicians for cover against claims for malpraxis may be as much as 100 times greater than premiums in the UK.

ACCESSIBILITY AND AVAILABILITY

Full availability of medical services is not uniform. Many areas and districts have shortages of services because physicians will not work in areas that may be geographically, economically or socially unattractive. There is no 'direction' or 'control' over the physicians.

'Free choice' of physician by patient is unreal in these under-doctored areas. It exists only in cities where most physicians choose to work and where there is a relative surfeit of medical resources.

THE MEDICAL PROFESSION

The medical profession in the USA is a strong and independent professional group.

Ethics and standards are in the hands of the various Colleges, Boards and Associations and medical politics has been the main concern and activity of the American Medical Association.

Currently there are major problems and stresses concerning the relations between the medical profession and the Federal and State authorities, particularly over the implications of Medicare and Medicaid; between the profession and the public as evident by the high level of medico-legal claims; between the profession and paramedical bodies over the demarcation disputes as to who should do what; and between various groups within the profession itself.

TABLE 5

Medical resources in the USA

Population	200 million
Physicians	297,000
	15 per 10,000 population
Annual number of new	7,500
medical graduates	4 per 100,000 population
Nurses	32 per 10,000 population
Paramedical workers	10 per 10,000 population
Hospital beds	8·9 per 1,000 population

(Sources: US Bureau of the Census, *U.S.A. 1967*, and *Health Manpower*, US Dept. HEW, 1967.)

The Structure of the Health Services in the UK

PRINCIPLES

1. In the United Kingdom a '*Welfare State*' has evolved. Within this the National Health Service (NHS) is the organ by which medical care is provided. Welfare and social services are organised by other government departments. The NHS is a 'new' service with an 'old' structure and resources and historically it has emerged from a mixture of National Health Insurance and private medical services.

2. Under the terms of the NHS medical care is free to the patient at the time of service.

3. Medical services are readily available and accessible to all.

4. Personal care is based on *generalist* first-contact services and on *specialist* hospital services.

5. Preventive care is accepted as important and worth while, but wholesale development of mass screening and pre-symptomatic checks has been delayed until there is more proof of their real place and value.

6. Community care, i.e. care of patients in their homes

and in the community outside hospitals, has been emphasised and is well developed.

7. Overall co-ordinated planning has been difficult because of the tripartite administrative structure of the NHS.

BASIC STRUCTURE

The British National Health Service still has a tripartite administrative structure in spite of the fact that there is a national Department of Health and Social Services with overall financial and administrative responsibilities, but with few opportunities for direct executive action.

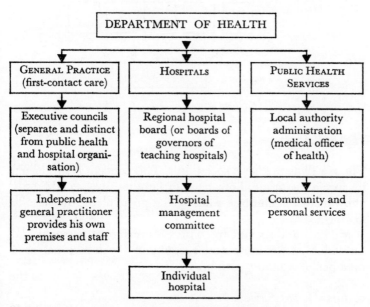

Fig. 5. Structure of UK medical services.

For various medico-political reasons it was not possible to alter the traditional partition of medical services into hospital, public health and general practice sectors in 1948 when the NHS was established.

Fig. 5 depicts the structure of medical services under the NHS.

Structure and Patterns of Medical Services

Within this tripartite administrative structure there are links between the various levels of care and the flow of care proceeds reasonably smoothly.

This *flow of care* is shown in Fig. 6.

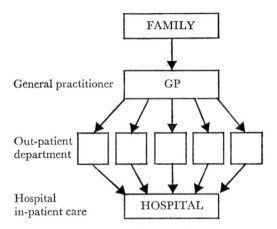

Fig. 6. Flow of medical care in the UK.

1. *The Family*

The family is the basic social unit. This concept is supported by special taxation allowances for families, by special family allowances for children and by the principle of the 'family doctor'.

Medical and social care, whilst it aims to be personal and individual, takes note and account of the individual as a member of a family group.

2. *First-Contact Services*

The general practitioner, or the family doctor, is the single medical portal of entry under the NHS. All citizens can 're-gister' as the patients of a general practitioner who is responsible for the medical care of all those who have registered with him. Each general practitioner cares for some 2,500 persons.

Patients have direct access to their general practitioner who is their sole regular doctor-of-first-contact.

General practitioners are independent and as a rule work from their own premises and employ their own staff.

Remuneration is through a combination of capitation fees for each person registered with the physician plus other payments for services such as obstetric work; preventive measures, such as immunisation and cervical cytology; night calls; reimbursement of salaries of staff and rates; and extra pay for working in a group of three or more physicians, for seniority and for special vocational training.

There is complete freedom of choice of doctor, by the patient, in his selection of whom he will register with.

Although the great majority (97 per cent) of the population is registered with a general practitioner it is quite possible, for any who seek it, to receive private care outside the NHS from a physician who wishes to provide such care.

A general practitioner in contract with the NHS may also engage in private paid work for persons who are not registered with him.

Working alongside, and often together with, general practitioners are public health nurses (health visitors), home nurses and district midwives employed by the local authority public health services. (See Chapter 6.)

3. *Out-patient Department*

Apart from accidents, emergencies or venereal diseases, access to the specialist services for ambulatory patients is only through the patient's general practitioner.

When he considers specialist advice or care is required the general practitioner refers his patients with a letter of introduction to the specialist clinics that are sited at the local hospital out-patient departments.

Almost all out-patient services are at NHS hospitals and are provided by highly trained and experienced specialists.

Specialists can also engage in private practice, but this accounts for less than 10 per cent of all specialist referrals.

4. *Hospital Services*

In addition to the out-patient specialist services for ambulatory cases NHS hospitals provide almost all of the beds and associated facilities for those requiring admission to hospital. Admission to hospital is either through the out-patient waiting list, directly through the general practitioner, or as an emergency via the hospital's casualty (emergency) unit.

Hospital senior medical staff are all specialists appointed on a competitive basis. General practitioners do not have access to hospital beds to treat their own patients – except in a few smaller and rural hospitals and in some obstetric units.

Pathological and radiological facilities are directly available to general practitioners for investigating their own patients. District hospitals also act as the local medical centre for education and research.

5. *Community Services*

Socio-medical services are provided through the health departments of the local authorities.

These services include home nursing, health education, home helps (for assistance with domestic duties), ambulance services and special services for the elderly, the handicapped and the mentally sick.

6. *Public Involvement*

Voluntary services such as the Red Cross, St John's, Royal Women's Voluntary Services and others are still active everywhere in spite of the NHS and the Welfare State.

ADMINISTRATION

The NHS was introduced in 1948 to provide a comprehensive health service available to all who need medical care. Apart from certain payments for dental care, eye glasses and a token contribution for prescriptions, all services are provided free of charge.

1. *The Department of Health and Social Security*

The Department of Health is responsible for the overall administration of the NHS in England and Wales. There are separate Departments of Health for Scotland and Northern Ireland.

The administrative head is a Member of Parliament, and appointed to take responsibility for the Department of Health. He is a professional politician and only once in the last fifty years has he been a physician.

The administrative head has direct responsibility for provision of hospital and specialist services, conduct of research (through the Medical Research Council), public health laboratory service and the blood transfusion service. He has indirect responsibility for general practitioner and local authority services.

At the Department he has a staff of full-time physicians and lay administrators and is advised also by a Central Health Services Council and standing expert advisory committees on various subjects.

The powers of the Department may appear great, but in practice its influence on medical practice depends on its relations with the medical profession and its ability through democratic means to persuade the profession to accept its proposals, and on good liaison with each of the three parts of the service involved in providing the actual medical care.

2. *Hospitals*

Hospital and specialist services are administered through 15 Regional Hospital Boards (RHB) and locally through Hospital Management Committees (HMC). Teaching hospitals are administered by Boards of Governors. Each RHB is associated with a medical school.

The 36 medical schools are not under the control of the Department of Health. Medical Schools are all a part of a local university which is responsible for the provision of teaching. The Department of Health, however, has the responsibility for providing the clinical facilities for the training of medical students.

3. *General Practice*

The administration of general medical (general practice) dental, pharmaceutical and optical services is through 134 Executive Councils. There is no geographical or other correspondence between the Executive Councils, the RHBs or public health divisions. Executive Councils have no planning powers. Planning of general medical care has been left to independent physicians, dentists, pharmacists and opticians.

The chief duties of Executive Councils are payment of

those providing services, dealing with complaints and advising consumers and providers on various details of the system.

4. *Public Health Services (Local Health Authorities)*

Public health services are administered by 175 elected councils of counties and boroughs.

The executive officer of these councils is the Medical Officer of Health who is a physician and a full-time employee of the local council.

BUDGETING

The NHS receives funds largely through direct and indirect taxation and to a lesser extent from direct payments arising from prescription costs, etc., and the monies paid for the use of 'private' and amenity hospital beds. The Department of Health prepares a budget which is provided by the Treasury after approval by Parliament.

Disimbursement is through the three parts of the service, namely the Regional Hospital Boards, the Executive Councils and the Local Health Authorities.

The NHS in 1966 accounted for 4·85 per cent of the gross

TABLE 6

Proportions of costs and sources of finance in the NHS in England and Wales

Proportions of expenditure in the NHS	
	%
Hospitals	60·9
General medical (general practice) services	7·5
Pharmaceuticals	11·2
General dental services	5·2
Supplementary ophthalmic costs	1·5
Local health authority (public health)	10·2
Other	3·5
Sources of monies for the NHS	
	%
Central exchequer (taxes)	72
NHS contributions (insurance)	12
Direct payments by consumers	4
Rates and grants from local authorities	12

(Source: Annual Report of Ministry of Health for 1966.)

national product (GNP), and this represented one-ninth of all public expenditure.

(The proportions of expenditure accounted for by the various services and the sources of the monies are shown in Table 6.)

In addition to the NHS costs there is a small amount of private practice in the UK and a number of hospital insurance schemes whereby those hospitalised are entitled to cover for private rooms and specialists' fees. Some 2 per cent of the population contribute to such schemes.

PLANNING

Although the NHS has resulted in a more tidy system of medical care and has made medical care available to all irrespective of ability to pay, planning has not resulted in any dramatic changes in the traditional structure of medical services in the UK.

In spite of many National Reports, Committees, Commissions and Recommendations, the tripartite organisation existing today is not very different from that prior to 1948.

Overall co-ordinated planning of all medical and social services has not been possible at either national, regional, district or local neighbourhood levels.

QUALITY CONTROLS

Maintenance of quality of care is still largely and traditionally a professional responsibility. There is no general and reliable system of built-in quality checks, although under the NHS it is possible for consumers to register complaints on any part of the medical or social service they have received, which can be investigated administratively.

AVAILABILITY, ACCESSIBILITY AND CHOICE

Accessibility has never been a problem in the UK since it is a small and densely populated island. Communications are good and all medical services are readily available in all areas.

MEDICAL PROFESSION

The British medical profession has long and ancient traditions with highly developed ethical and professional standards.

The introduction of the NHS has not altered these standards nor interfered with professional independence and freedom. The many and various professional bodies, colleges, associations and academies, are completely free to organise their work and activities without any interference from the State.

What the NHS has produced is an employment monopoly. Almost all practising physicians are in contract with the NHS and such a monopoly has inevitably resulted in occasional differences between profession and State on rates of remuneration and terms of service.

Negotiations on such medico-political matters are largely in the hands of the British Medical Association but in more professional and academic matters there is no single recognisable and accepted leadership, each college and association represents only those who belong to it and there is no one professional body to speak for all.

RESOURCES

The current medical resources are shown in Table 7.

TABLE 7

Medical resources in England and Wales

Population	50 million
Physicians	55,000
	11 per 10,000 population
Annual number of new	1,600
medical graduates	3·2 per 100,000 population
Nurses	35 per 10,000 population
Paramedical workers	10 per 10,000 population
Hospital beds	10·1 per 1,000 population

(Source: Annual Report of Ministry of Health for 1966.)

Comparisons

Some general comparisons may be made at this stage – more detailed ones will emerge in dealing with specific topics.

BASIC STRUCTURE AND PROBLEMS

With similar challenges to provide high quality medical care for developed societies each of the three nations is faced with certain specific problems related to national factors.

The USSR has developed an impressive system of medical care that is available and accessible to all. It has created tremendous resources of medical personnel, trained and in training, but there are problems relating to the fundamental structure.

In a service that has had to be built from almost nothing in fifty years there was bound to be rigidity and standardisation of planning control. This persists and there is such a degree of uniformity in this monolithic structure of the Soviet system that lack of resilience, difficulties in self-evaluation and criticism, inability for new ideas and methods in providing medical care to be tried out, are apparent; and there are few incentives and little encouragement for the more peripheral medical workers to become involved in the formulation of new ideas and experiments.

Having built up a system designed to meet needs and stresses of the past, one might question how the Soviet system will achieve flexibility and devolution to meet the inevitable changing social and medical customs of the future.

In the USA the problems of medical care are different. In a wealthy nation with a philosophy of free enterprise, self-help and self-responsibility for medical care, high quality of medical care has become customary for those able to pay for it. The challenge facing the USA however, is how to make such care available to all who need it, and particularly the under-privileged. They, face the challenge, and difficulty, of redeploying their resources to meet the needs of the whole population and it is not certain how the medical profession, the State, and the public will react to this.

In the UK the problems are different yet again, but they are also those of change and readjustment. Not only is there need for an old and traditional system to readjust itself to a new concept of a welfare society, but this change in medical care is taking place in the wider context of an international political shift. The UK is having to alter its role in the world of nations from a global to a continental power and is facing the challenge of actually being able to afford, what politically and publicly it wants from its medical services.

Common to the three nations is the problem of implementing changes. It is a situation that is bound up with difficulties of national and professional leadership, decisions, actions and achievements.

FAMILY AND FIRST-CONTACT CARE

Whilst the family is the basic social unit in the USSR, the USA and the UK, the concept of a single 'family doctor' is strong only in the UK and this may be merely an unintentional effect of the 'freezing' of the old form of medical care in 1948 into the three parts – general practice (family medicine), hospital and public health services.

In the USA where there has been freedom to develop trends and fashions, first-contact care is carried out by a series of 'specialoids', namely, paediatricians, internists and others who confine their work to certain age or disease groups. However, this trend in the USA towards specialisation at this first-contact level seems to have been effected more by professional than consumer forces. The average American family seems to yearn for the 'good old family doctor' of their past memories.

In the USSR it was decided and decreed in the 1930s that first-contact care was to be divided and that various members of the family would attend different physicians. This decision has resulted in a splintering of first-contact services carried out, as it is in the USA, by a series of 'specialoids', i.e. local paediatricians, therapists and others, who often work from separate polyclinics and who rarely come together in dealing with family problems.

In the UK because of the structure of the NHS the doctor-of-first-contact is a 'generalist'. He cares for all the diseases and problems of a mixed and undifferentiated population of all ages and both sexes. He is the single portal of entry for his patients into the British system of medical care.

An emotional debate is going on as to which system is

more suitable for modern needs – the single-portal of entry generalist type of British 'family doctor' or the Soviet or American type 'specialoid'?

No reliable comparative studies have been made, neither to measure quality and efficacy, nor to assess the views of the public.

AMBULATORY SPECIALIST SERVICES

Different patterns exist in each of the three countries. In the UK there is a rigid system of highly developed hospital-based specialist out-patient departments to whom referral is only through the general practitioner.

In the USSR these specialist services work from community centred polyclinics that in most urban areas are distinct and separate from local hospitals, even to the extent of having different staffs.

In the USA the pattern is mixed with private practice, group practice, clinics and hospital out-patient departments each playing a part.

HOSPITALS

The structure of modern hospitals is similar in the three nations but there is a difference in the medical staffing.

In the USA it is customary for almost all local physicians to have access to some hospital beds. In the UK and the USSR hospital specialists are specially trained and appointed and the first-contact physicians do not have access to hospital beds in which they may treat their patients.

ADMINISTRATION

There is a range from the rigidly monolithic administrative structure of the USSR with ultimate overall controls in the Ministry of Health of the USSR and neat organisational structure at various geographical levels, through the system in the UK where control is possible in theory by the Department of Health but where the degrees of actual power are limited in practice, and to the USA where recent changes are only now creating opportunities for central planning and administration.

E

RESOURCES

The resources in medical man- and woman-power in the USSR are greater in terms of physicians and paramedics than in the USA or the UK and in spite of this the output of physicians in the next five years in the USSR is being almost doubled.

TABLE 8

Comparison of resources

	USSR	USA	UK
Population	230 million	200 million	50 million
Physicians	550,000	297,000	55,000
	1 per 415	1 per 710	1 per 900
	24 per 10,000	15 per 10,000	11 per 10,000
Annual number of new	30,000	7,500	1,600
medical graduates	12 per 100,000	4 per 100,000	3·2 per 100,000
Nurses	35 per 10,000	32 per 10,000	35 per 10,000
Paramedical workers	37 per 10,000	10 per 10,000	10 per 10,000
Hospital beds	9.6 per 1,000	8·9 per 1,000	10·1 per 1,000

What do these differences mean?

There are a number of possibilities which must be speculative until reliable and fair comparisons by planned studies can be undertaken.

It may mean that the needs of the USSR for physicians are greater to control and manage a higher rate of morbidity – this is doubtful because although certain indices of social progress such as the incidence of tuberculosis and rheumatic fever are somewhat higher in the USSR, the standards of health in the three nations judged by other health measures, are comparable. It may be that new roles are foreseen for physicians in the expansion of preventive and health educational services, but the true value of such efforts are still unproven. It may be that there is gross under-utilisation and misuse of Soviet physicians. The work-load and work-schedules of Soviet physicians are geared to a 6½-hour day and a 5-day week, and the norms of work show that compared with British and American physicians the numbers of patients seen are less although the demands from the consumers are greater. (See Chapter 4.)

MEDICAL PROFESSION

The independent, professional and academic status of the physician has been replaced in the USSR by that of a necessary, but not over-privileged, member of society. She (for 70 per cent of physicians are women) has her place in the social hierarchy that is equal to that of other skilled and professional groups, for example the engineers, teachers and scientists, and the Soviet medical professional organisations are similar to those of other professional groups, fulfilling a trade union role rather than an academic and professional role.

Whether such a situation affects the ultimate quality of medical care or the satisfaction of the physician is uncertain.

Chapter 4
First Contact Care

In all systems of medical care all over the world there is a doctor-of-first-contact, *a primary physician, who exercises similar roles and functions. The ways in which this first-contact care is organised will differ in each system but the broad principles are the same.*

This physician is the first medically qualified person seen by the patient in times of medical need and this doctor-of-first-contact lives and works in a relatively static community of limited and small size.

The physician will encounter all grades of disease as they occur naturally, but because 'common diseases commonly occur and rare diseases rarely happen' the primary physician's work will be largely with the fortunately trivial and less serious types of disease.

The physician in this field of medical care often provides long-term and continuing care, and he must have aid and assistance from a wide range of paramedical workers such as nurses, socio-medical assistants and clerical aides.

He acts as the primary medical assessor of the patient and his medical needs, and he acts as a protective screen for the hospitals.

Working as he does in a community where he is well known and respected this doctor has good opportunities to undertake preventive care and health education in a personal sense during each of his consultations. He is also in a good position to know and study the special local social epidemiological and clinical problems of his small community and to carry out studies to define possible remediable factors.

The USSR

First contact care in the USSR incorporates all of the principles on which Soviet medical care is based. The care provided is free, there is ready and direct access to the service, the physicians who work in this field are 'specialoids', preventive measures occupy a large part of the work and there is encouragement for public self-help involvement.

There are other notable features. There is no free choice of doctor. Geographical boundaries define the physician's zone of work and persons living within the specified area are allocated to that physician' These defined neighbourhood areas are termed uchastoks and doctors-of-first-contact are referred to as *uchastok* (or local) *physicians*.

THE PLACE OF THE DOCTOR-OF-FIRST-CONTACT

The principle of the primary physician providing direct access and continuing personal care for the patient is fully accepted in the USSR.

Since all physicians in the USSR are recognised as 'specialists' this belief also applies to first-contact care. Specialisation is attempted everywhere, except in the more remote rural areas, through sharing of primary care between a local paediatrician, who provides care for children up to 15 years of age, a local therapist (internist), who looks after the medical ills of adults, a local dental surgeon and a local occupational physician in industrial regions.

Division of primary medical care between separate physicians is a basic feature. There is no place at present for the 'generalist' in the Soviet system.

Local physicians work from polyclinics with nurses and feldshers (middle grade medical workers), but in the polyclinics there are also specialists to whom patients may be referred by these physicians and to whom patients also have direct access.

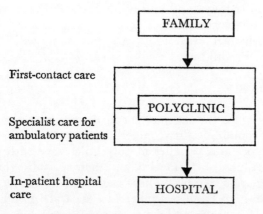

Fig. 7. First-contact care in the USSR.

First Contact Care

The *District hospital* in any area is distinct from the poly-clinic. It has its own separate medical staff and although there are exchanges of less senior staff the local physicians do not have access to hospital beds, except in rural areas.

The polyclinic combines primary first-contact care with ambulatory specialist services and that there is sharing of first-contact care between paediatric, therapeutic (adult internal medicine), dental and occupational physicians.

THE 'UCHASTOK' PRINCIPLE

The principle of local geographical division is not con-fined to first-contact care. It is a useful administrative pro-cedure of ensuring cover and responsibility for the commun-ity services of a population of about 4,000 in the care of tuberculosis, the provision of maternity services, the care of mental illness and the organisation of public health ser-vices.

The *uchastok* physicians do not work as a closely knit harmonious unit. In larger urban communities each of the four main 'specialoid' sub-groups may be attached to a separate polyclinic. Thus, the paediatrician may work from a children's polyclinic, the therapist from an adult poly-clinic, the dentist from a dental polyclinic and the occupa-tional physician from an industrial medical unit.

Family care based on a single polyclinic, a comprehensive local team or a family physician is not evident.

In smaller towns and villages, because of the small popu-lation, one physician does combine occupational medical care and hygiene with adult care, but rarely will he or she also care for children.

POLYCLINICS

Polyclinics are the primary medical units within the com-munity, combining first-contact and specialist services.

The types and varieties of polyclinics vary with the size and geography of the locality and their specialist roles.

In *large cities* splintering has occurred. In Moscow, Lenin-grad and other large cities there are separate polyclinics for children, for adults, and for disease entities such as women's diseases, tuberculosis, mental illnesses, dental surgery and skin and venereal diseases.

In *small cities* there is generally a single all-purpose poly-clinic that provides care for the whole local population, but within such a clinic there is separation of children, adults and various disease categories amongst different physicians.

No trend is notable towards centralising and co-ordinat-ing services for the care of the whole family in one poly-clinic by a single team. Distinct services exist for child care with a set of paediatricians, separate from physicians, who care for father and mother. Father, mother or child may be under the care of three or more physicians in separate buildings at the same time.

The populations served by polyclinics depend on the loca-lity. In large cities an adult polyclinic may serve a popula-tion of from 40,000 to 60,000 adults and a children's poly-clinic may provide care in the same and corresponding section of the city for between 15,000 and 20,000 children under the age of 15. One women's consultation clinic on the other hand may cover a number of such areas and provide care for up to 250,000 women.

THE WORK OF THE LOCAL PHYSICIAN

The population of an average *uchastok* will be 4,000 persons and the following physicians will be involved:

A Paediatrician will care for 700–1,200 children under 15.
A Therapist will care for 2,000 adults.
An Occupational physician will care for 1,000–2,000 workers. (Care of these will be shared with the thera-pist.)
A Dental surgeon will care for 2,000 persons.

The *nature of the work* of the local physician is similar to that of first-contact physicians in the USA and the UK, with two important differences.

First, much of the work in the Soviet polyclinics is for preventive purposes, and it is reported that one-half of the average ten annual attendances per person at polyclinics are for 'preventive examinations'.

Second, overt emotional disorders appear to be infrequent, and the mass of clinical work is with common respiratory, digestive and rheumatic conditions.

The *methods of work* are through consultations at the polyclinic and home visits to the patients' homes.

Home visits are encouraged rather than discouraged and sick children are unwelcome at polyclinics. Prominent notices advise parents to call the physician to their homes when their child is sick. It is customary for a nurse or feldsher to accompany the physician on home visits.

In addition to regular clinical work, local physicians are involved actively in health education and preventive activities in the dispenserisation scheme.

The *volume of work* undertaken by the local physicians is regulated by established and agreed norms and standards, and all physicians have a 5-day week of $6\frac{1}{2}$–7 hours per day, with a maximum of 35 hours work per week.

A '*day*' comprises one consulting session and one home visiting session. Each session is planned to last about 3 hours.

At her polyclinic consulting session the local paediatrician or therapist expects to see 15 patients during 3 hours, allowing each patient some 12 minutes of the physician's time.

Each home visit averages half an hour, including travel in a chauffeur-driven car, so that 6 home visits will be carried out each day.

In addition to this work the physician sets aside $\frac{1}{2}$–1 hour each day for health education through talks, lectures, demonstrations or some other means.

Physician-cover for emergency and night work is through a rota. In the larger polyclinics there is a separate staff on call for such purposes.

THE 'UCHASTOK' PHYSICIANS

The great majority, 80 per cent, of local, or neighbourhood, physicians are women (70 per cent of *all* physicians in the USSR are women).

There is no special vocational training for this work. Following the standard medical education (see Chapter 12) the graduate physician may apply for, or be directed to, work in a polyclinic. To begin she will work under the guidance and supervision of more senior colleagues.

Career progression depends on seniority and merit, and there are many opportunities for advancement through post-graduate education, study and examination. Remuneration is related to seniority and merit.

ACCESS AND AVAILABILITY

There is no free choice of physician. Persons within a geographical neighbourhood are allocated to that physician who has been assigned for the particular locality.

If, as sometimes happens, doctor–patient relations become strained and difficult, then it is possible for the patient (or doctor) to be allocated to an alternative physician (or patient).

There is direct access by the patient to the physician. Appointments at polyclinics are unusual but because of the small numbers seen in any session there apparently are no unduly long waits.

URBAN AND RURAL DIFFERENCES

To provide a full and accessible service in rural as well as in urban situations requires considerable adaptation to local problems. The provision of medical care in rural areas is made more difficult because of the smaller and more widely dispersed populations and the distances involved, and it is not practically possible to provide physicians for every small and outlying community.

A compromise has been achieved in the USSR whereby paramedical workers, such as nurses, midwives and socio-medical workers (feldshers), provide some of the first-contact

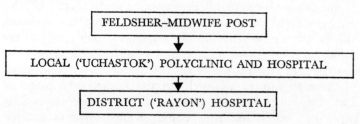

Fig. 8. Structure of medical care in rural USSR.

care in collaboration with, and supervised by, physicians from polyclinics and hospitals.

The primary units of medical care in rural areas (and more than half of the USSR is classified as 'rural') are the feldsher–midwife post and the combined local polyclinic and hospital. (Fig. 8.)

FELDSHER–MIDWIFE POST

These are medical and nursing units normally staffed by a feldsher (*vide infra*) and a midwife. In some units there is a single feldsher–midwife combining the two roles. Sited in remote rural areas often 20 or even 100 miles from the local polyclinic and hospital these units provide personal and continuing care for populations varying from a hundred to a few thousands. Care is organised for minor ailments routine preventive medical work and supervision of hygiene, and sanitation is an important duty. Anything other than minor ailments are referred to the physician either at the polyclinic or she is asked to call and visit the patient at home.

Such units are all under the supervision of a local physician based at the polyclinic–hospital who may have a number of such units to supervise. The physician visits each unit at regular intervals of 2–4 weeks and is always available for emergencies.

The feldsher is a traditional Russian character. Originally a second-class doctor introduced into the Russian armies in the eighteenth century and later to the peasant communities to meet shortages of physicians, the feldsher is now a qualified middle-grade paramedical worker who has undergone a special three-year training course and who no longer works alone but in co-operation with, and under the supervision of, a physician.

Although chiefly found in the rural areas of the USSR, feldshers also work in more specialised fields in urban communities such as emergency care (ambulance attendants), tuberculosis, mental illness and occupational health and preventive care, as medical social workers.

Although almost all births in the USSR take place in maternity units there is still a place for *district midwives* who carry out ante-natal supervision. Such midwives receive special training and in rural areas work together with the feldsher (in very remote places there is a feldsher–midwife who combines the work). They all work under the supervision of the obstetrician from the local (*uchastok*) hospital.

UCHASTOK POLYCLINIC–HOSPITAL

In rural areas the polyclinic and hospital are combined in a single unit. Serving a population of between 5,000 and 15,000 the unit is staffed by a group of physicians and nurses, and the medical staff comprises primary physicians and general specialists, who may include surgeons, obstetricians, radiologists, dentists and others, depending on the size of the population cared for.

Each of the local physicians has her neighbourhood area that includes a number of feldsher–midwife posts for which she is responsible.

Mobile units for dental and preventive care, including a mobile miniature radiography unit are based on the local polyclinic–hospital. They visit collective farms and villages regularly to provide on-the-spot care for the people.

There is close communication between these hospitals and the District hospitals, and specialists from these larger units often come out by road or air transport for consultations or to carry out special therapeutic procedures.

SOLO OR GROUP?

The 'solo-generalist' physician has disappeared from the Soviet medical system. Even in the most remote rural areas first-contact care is provided through groups of local physicians in contact with feldshers and working closely with specialists.

The specialist sub-divisions of '*uchastok*' physicians into paediatricians and therapists has been noted and so has the allocations of populations in neighbourhood areas. There is now a move to group together 4 or 5 of these local physicians so that the therapists would care for up to 10,000 persons, and paediatricians for up to 5,000 children. There is, however, no intention of grouping together therapists and paediatricians to act as a family group.

HEALTH TEAM

The local or neighbourhood physicians work closely with

65

paramedical auxiliaries. Each physician has a *nurse* working with her. This nurse is an all-purpose worker who combines receptionist and clerical duties with nursing. She receives and prepares patients for the physician in the polyclinic and she assists in record-keeping. She carries out standard nursing tasks in the polyclinic and accompanies the physician on some home visits and carries out others for follow-up or for preventive measures alone. The paediatric nurse is much involved in well-baby care both in the polyclinic and on home visits to the young mother.

Modern office techniques are absent from the polyclinics. Most records and letters would seem to be handwritten and there are few typewriters and hardly any data-processing machines in spite of the mass of records that have to be analysed for statistical purposes. Sorting and analysis at the polyclinic level is, in the main, carried out by hand by clerical staff.

Feldshers who work in urban polyclinics often act as medical social workers attached to specialities, for example in care of the tuberculous, the mentally ill, the chronic sick and handicapped, and are involved actively in health education and preventive care.

In rural areas feldshers act as the medical workers of first-contact to small and outlying communities.

FACILITIES AND RELATIONS WITH OTHER SERVICES

Diagnostic and therapeutic facilities are available for the local physicians.

Every polyclinic has radiological and pathological facilities, and although the scope of diagnostic work depends on the size of the polyclinic, nevertheless in each clinic straight radiographs and contrast-media radiology can be carried out.

The clinic's pathological laboratories are integrated with larger units at the District hospital and the local public health laboratory.

The *'uchastok'* physician has ready access to specialist advice from the specialists who are working in the same building and admissions of patients to hospital present few problems since there is no shortage of beds.

Social and welfare services are provided through the

Sanepid (public health) service, which is associated closely with all the polyclinics in its area.

UTILISATION

It has been estimated that 80 per cent of Soviet citizens attend their polyclinics every year, and further that the average annual attendance-rate is between 7 and 10 attendances per person at risk.

These attendances combine first-contact and specialist care, accident, emergency and dental services for ambulatory patients.

A break-down of the expected (the standard norm) annual number of attendances per person at a polyclinic is shown in Table 9.

Of particular note are the low proportions of attendances for 'neurology and psychiatry' and the high rate for tuberculosis, whilst also included are 2·0 attendances for dental care (from a dental surgeon), although such attendances would not be included in the work load of similar units in the USA and the UK.

TABLE 9

Norms for annual attendances per person at polyclinics in the USSR

General medical	2·5
General surgical	1·4
Paediatric	1·3
OBG (obstetrics and gynaecology)	0·8
Eyes	0·5
ENT	0·4
Neurology and psychiatry	0·4
Tuberculosis	0·3
Skin and VD	0·4
Dental	2·0
TOTAL	10·0

Attendances for 'preventive examinations' amounting to 5·0 are included in the various sections.
(Source: Popov, G.A. *The Efficiency of Medical Care*, WHO, EURO, *294*, 2, 1967.)

The USA

There is no set type of primary physician in the USA. The nature and pattern of first-contact care depends on geography and locale, on social class and income and on local customs and traditions.

The spectrum ranges from the old-type family general practitioner, who is still to be found in the smaller mid-Western communities, through specialoid paediatricians and internists to the most highly specialised groups of Clinic physicians in New York and Los Angeles.

Recent legislation that has resulted in the implementation of Medicare and Medicaid services is nevertheless creating changes in the patterns of first-contact care, by making such care available to many unable to afford it before. However, these changes have not yet altered the broad patterns of care.

THE PLACE OF THE DOCTOR-OF-FIRST-CONTACT

The American patient has the choice of multiple portals of entry into the system of medical care at the first-contact level.

It is often left to the patient to choose and select (where he can) the physician that he, the patient, considers appropriate to the presenting situation. In large cities as New York it is not unusual for a family to 'shop around' the local medical profession and utilise a large number of primary physicians.

The *primary physician* may be one of many types.

1. The *Hospital Emergency Room* provides first-contact care for local poor and indigent community in larger American cities. This service has developed over many years to make available a form of medical care for those unable to meet the fees of a personal private physician.

Physicians who staff the hospital emergency rooms are often young, newly qualified and medically immature, seeking to gain medical experience. They genuinely seek to provide good medical care for their patients, but it is impossible for this care to be anything but *ad hoc*, discontinuous and episodic.

2. The *Solo-generalist physician*, the old type 'do-it-all-

yourself' general practitioner, who cares for patients of all ages and for all their presenting conditions, including some surgery, obstetrics and child care, is becoming rare. He is still to be found in the smaller and outlying communities. In the larger cities of the USA there are, however, physicians who believe in 'family medicine' and combine paediatrics with internal medicine in their practice.

Nevertheless there is an increasing public demand for the return of the family doctor, a physician of high quality who is able to care for the whole family at the first-contact level and who makes no pretence to be a restrictive specialist.

3. The *'Specialoid'*. In larger cities first-contact care has been divided between paediatricians and internists, who restrict their work to specific age-groups – children up to 15 years, or to certain specified internal medical ailments of adults. It is a truism that the doctor-of-first-contact in any system inevitably cares for the common and less serious disorders in his relatively small and static community and he cannot expect to become experienced in the treatment of the rarer and more serious diseases.

Paediatricians and internists who provide first-contact care are unlikely to become specialists, in the true sense, because of such limitations of experience. They must therefore be considered as 'specialoids'.

4. The *Specialist*. Direct access by the patient to a recognised specialist, who has attained certification by specialist boards, is customary in the USA.

Much of the work of dermatologists, neurologists, gynaecologists, general surgeons, ophthalmologists and even neuro-surgeons, is of the patient self-referral character. In addition these specialists see patients referred to them by other medical colleagues. The proportion of these two types of patients, the self-referred and the colleague-referred, depends on the seniority and the attitudes of the specialist. The more senior specialist will attract a higher proportion of colleague-referred patients than will a young specialist seeking as much work as possible. Specialists who accept self-referred patients are prepared also to undertake more general continuing care, often outside their speciality, for these patients. In this way they combine the role of a primary physician with that of a specialist.

The pattern and nature of the work of the primary physician in the USA depends on his type. The work of the young physician in the emergency room will be very different from that of the internist or of a general practitioner. The former is faced with more dramatic situations in the later stages of diseases affecting the indigent poor, whereas the private primary physician will be concentrating more on the early stages of disease and on prevention and presymptomatic diagnosis.

The population cared for by the primary physician varies considerably because of the mobility of the population (it has been estimated that one family in five moves home annually in the USA), the mobility of physician and because it is not traditional to remain constantly under the care of one physician. It is therefore not unusual for patients to be under the care of more than one physician at the same time. Tables 10 and 11 demonstrate the common morbidity

TABLE 10

Annual expected disease prevalence per 1,000 at risk in general practice, in the USA

	Rates per 1,000 at risk
Acute	
Upper respiratory infections	305
Minor accidents	56
Acute skin infections	31
Acute bronchitis and pneumonia	7
Appendicitis	3
Chronic	
Emotional problems	40
Chronic skin disorders	20
High blood pressure	25
Peptic ulcers	10
Asthma	11
New growths	3
Diabetes	6

(Source: Huntley, R.R. (1963). *J. Amer. Med. Assoc.*, *185*, 175. Quoting data from the New York Health Insurance Plan Groups, 1948–1951).

TABLE 11

'Top 10' disorders in general practice in the USA, in rates per 1,000 of visits to physicians

		Per 1,000 visits to physcian
1.	Upper respiratory infections	75
2.	Bronchitis and 'flu	37
3.	High blood pressure	28
4.	Coronary heart disease	25
5.	Obesity	22
6.	Arthritis	18
7.	Diabetes	12
8.	Menopause	12
9.	Anaemia	11
10.	Otitis media	11

(Source: Huntley, R.R. (1963). Evidence presented to Citizens Commission on Graduate Medical Education, quoting National Disease and Therapeutic Index Medical Report No. 6. 1962.)

patterns reported from a number of US practices and they confirm that the American doctor-of-first-contact is dealing with the more common disorders, as in fact, do his colleagues elsewhere in the world.

Showing the variation in the nature of work between the general practitioner, internist and paediatrician in the USA, Table 12 emphasises the special nature of the work of the three. Namely, that the paediatrician is concerned principally with well-child care and minor upper respiratory infections, the GP with a broad range of diseases and the

TABLE 12

Nature of work of paediatrician, GP and internist in the USA, in relation to certain diseases and expressed in rates per 100 patient visits

Diseases per 100 patient visits	Paediatrician	GP	Internist
Cardiovascular diseases	0	6	18
Upper respiratory tract infections	22	10	4
Bronchitis and pneumonia	3	3	2
Prophylactic procedures	31	15	9

(Source: Adapted from White, K.L. (1964). *J. Med. Educ.*, *39*, 333.)

internist with degenerative disorders and medical check-ups.

The American primary physicians organise their work through consultations at their office, with visits to homes and hospitals. Access to hospital beds is a special feature of first-contact care in the USA.

In the Health Insurance Plan of New York (HIP) in 1965 the work was apportioned as follows:

Office consultations	Home visits	Hospital visits
84 per cent	4 per cent	12 per cent

It is noted in this report for 1965 that the rate of home visiting had decreased by more than one half during the preceding decade. There has been an active and successful policy by physicians in the USA to reduce home visiting to a minimum. Inevitably this policy has created friction between patients and physicians for patients have resented being forced to travel to clinic, office or hospital when sick.

VOLUME OF WORK

The volume of work carried out by the American physician varies considerably, and whilst some may work 60 hours or more a week, others may spend less than 20 hours in their professional work. No quoted studies can cover the whole range.

A study carried out by Kroeger et al. (1966), on internists in New York, found that the internists studied saw 85 patients in a week and spent 35–40 hours at work (Table 13).

TABLE 13

Work pattern of internists in New York

	Consulta-tions	Home visits	Hospital visits	Total items of work	Time spent (hours)
A week	55	5	25	85	35–40
A day	11	1	5	17	7–8
Per cent	65%	6%	29%	—	—

(Source: Kroeger, H.H., et al. (1965). J. Amer. Med. Assoc., 193, 371–376, 667–672, 916–922; 194, 177–81, 553–538.)

According to T.S. Eimerl (1967) (NZ Med. J., 66, 15) the work-load of a general practitioner in the USA in 1953/

54 at 165 items or work per week, was double that of the internists quoted.

There is free choice of physician in the USA, but access to private physicians depends on the patients ability to meet their fees.

Availability depends on locale and the ratio of physicians to population. Thus in outlying rural areas there may be no physicians available for many miles.

ORGANISATION

Most primary physicians in the USA work alone in competition with their colleagues. They may share common buildings with separate office suites but although partnerships and groupings are increasing they are still a minority, and it is estimated that only some 10–15 per cent of all primary physicians work in groups.

These groups include specialists and primary physicians sharing premises and who endeavour to provide total care for patients attending the group.

A few very large groups work from central buildings referred to as Clinics. One of the best known is the Mayo Clinic in Rochester, Minnesota, and this world-renowned Clinic comprises both first-contact and specialist ambulatory services. Its chief work however is in the specialist field, but it must be classed as providing a first-contact service, since 50–60 per cent of all patients who attend the Mayo Clinic are self-referred.

PREMISES AND EQUIPMENT

In general the standards of equipment and premises are high. Except in special situations such as in government-sponsored services and hospitals all the equipment is provided by and paid for by the physicians.

THE HEALTH TEAM

Primary physicians employ their own staff. This comprises nurses, secretaries and other assistants such as laboratory, radiological and physiotherapeutic ancillaries, and whilst these paramedical workers work entirely under the direction of the physicians, it is most unusual for them to act as first-contact workers, as do the Soviet feldshers.

An explanation for this is the fee-for-service system. When the patient pays the physician he does not expect to be treated by his nurse, he expects to be treated by the physician. Whilst midwives in the USSR and UK carry out most normal deliveries, in the USA there are few trained midwives and the physician is expected to carry out all normal obstetric procedures because it is not customary to share either the work or the fees. There are thus few links between primary physicians and the medical social workers and nursing staff employed by local community services.

CAREER STRUCTURE AND STATUS

No recognisable career structure has been developed for primary physicians in the USA because there are so many different types of physician carrying out these roles.

The American Academy of General Practice with 25,000 members has succeeded in 1969 in creating a Speciality Board for 'General Practice' and hopes to develop an acceptable training and career structure, but the chief problem is to attract young physicians into this field.

At present training is left to the individual. It is based on a hospital training with the goal of achieving board certification in some speciality such as internal medicine or paediatrics. Then, once in practice, the intention of the young doctor is usually to combine work in the specialist branch with first-contact care.

Primary physicians in the USA appear to be well satisfied with their work and income but uncertain of their exact roles. Their patients, however, are not so well satisfied with the care provided. They complain of over-specialisation, over-investigation, over-hospitalisation, over-charging and under-personalisation of care. They are unhappy because the physicians will not visit them at home and they speak with reminiscent affection of their old-type family doctors.

FACILITIES AND RELATIONS WITH OTHER SERVICES

The primary physician generally has good facilities for diagnosis and treatment, since they are provided either by the physician himself, or by specialist collegues who are in private radiological and pathological practice, or at local hospitals.

Diagnostic facilities: The solo physician may often possess his own radiological equipment operated by one of his ancillary staff, although contrast media radiography is usually referred to a specialist radiologist – alternatively physicians will refer all cases for radiography to such a colleague.

Pathological facilities likewise may be undertaken by the physician or referred to a private laboratory, for the primary physician, if he is working alone, cannot undertake more than simple and basic investigations in his own consulting suite.

Physicians working in groups or clinics endeavour to provide diagnostic facilities in their own premises.

Hospitals: Access to hospital beds is customary for the primary physician in the States. Such access, however, depends on the locale, and in the largest cities not all physicians have such access. Hospitals discriminate and accept only a proportion of physicians for full privileges, this acceptance depending on the skills, training and experience of the physician.

In smaller cities and rural areas full hospital privileges are usually available for all local physicians, but hospital committees have the right to deny such privileges.

There are considerable financial incentives for primary physicians in the USA to treat patients in hospitals. High fees can be charged, and since most of these are underwritten through pre-paid insurance schemes, neither physicians or patients are inhibited from hospitalisation.

Most insurance policies provide cover for care of patients who require hospitalisation but not for ambulatory treatment outside hospital and this may well account for the relatively high rates of hospitalisation in the USA. (See also Chapter 6.)

The limitation and restriction of types of cases treated, and procedures undertaken, by primary physicians varies with the hospital. Some hospitals limit, others restrict and yet others have no limitations. Special problems arise for example with surgical procedures. Since the fees charged for surgical procedures are high and much higher than for non-surgical care there are incentives and temptations for physicians to carry out surgical operations. In many hospitals in the USA primary physicians are entitled to carry out appendicectomies, cholecystectomies and hysterectomies, as well as less major operations such as removal of tonsils, ligature of varicose veins and repair of hernias.

In general, relations between primary physicians and welfare and public health services tend to be on a formal plane and no close co-operation between private medical and public community services has occurred.

UTILISATION

The US citizen makes between 4 and 5 visits to his physicians each year and between 1 and 2 visits to his dentist.

Thus the US Bureau of the Census (*USA 1967*) states that in 1963/64 the average number of visits to physicians were 4·5 (males 4·0 and females 5·1).

The Health Insurance Plan of New York states that during 1965 its 700,000 employees received 4·7 services from their physicians (males 4·5 and females 5·0). Over the longer period 1950–1965 the rates ranged from 4·7 to 5·2.

O.L. Peterson *et al.* (1967) (*Lancet, 1,* 771) quote that, based on household interviews in 1959, the physician utilisation rate was 5·3 attendances during the year.

The UK

The concept of the general practitioner who is also a 'family doctor' has been traditionally accepted as an essential feature of the British system of medical care. Agreement on this principle has led to the continuance of traditional and established patterns in spite of the advent of the new National Health Service (NHS) in 1948. Under the NHS it was decreed that 'general practice' was to persist as a distinct part with its own administrative structure.

It was accepted also that under the NHS all persons should have free access to a general practitioner, with whom they might register, and that he should act as a personal physician and as the main 'portal of entry' into the system of medical care.

THE PLACE OF THE DOCTOR-OF-FIRST-CONTACT

The traditional form of first-contact care in the UK for the past 400 years has been general practice. In the sixteenth and seventeenth centuries the Apothecaries were the first general practitioners. These 'physicians of the people' were distinct from the Surgeons and Physicians. Each of these three professional groups formed its own College or Society (in the case of Apothecaries), and each received royal charters and blessings from the Monarch of the time.

Always distinct from specialist and hospital practice, British general practice has been based on an independent and private entrepreneur system. Such a system still continues in the NHS with general practitioners working independently from their own premises, with their own staff and organising their work as they consider fit, meeting only the general criteria and safeguards set by the General Medical Council to ensure professional safeguards and standards.

The NHS, when introduced in 1948, created no new system of first-contact care, merely perpetuating set and existing patterns, and the same general practitioners continued to work from the same premises in the same ways as before. The concept of community health centres was not acceptable to the medical profession whose members opted to work in the established fashion.

A main financial feature of the new NHS was the abolition of fees for services and the extension of the capitation system, already in existence for certain workers, to the whole population. Now, in 1969, some 97 per cent of the population are registered with general practitioners.

Private practice was not prohibited, but with time the proportion of general practitioners engaged solely in private practice has fallen to 1 per cent of all those in practice and although many general practitioners may combine some private with their NHS work, very few receive more than 10 per cent of their income from private practice.

In the British NHS there is a complete free-choice of doctor and patient. Patients can 'register' with any general practitioner of their choosing, who, if he agrees to accept the patient, undertakes to provide all necessary and appropriate medical care. The physician is allowed to accept up to 3,500 patients. At present the average number of patients cared for by each general practitioner is 2,500.

The general practitioner functions as a generalist and provides first-level medical care to all those registered with him. He endeavours to provide personal and family care for an unbiased sample of the population, and does not restrict his work to any special age, sex, disease or system divisions.

He is, apart from emergencies, the main portal of entry into the British system of medical care. His patients have direct access to him and he provides long-term and continuing care for his patients. He sees almost three out of four of all his patients at least once a year and at least one member from 9 out of 10 of all families in his practice population each year. Since fewer than 10 per cent of British families move home in any one year, the general practitioner comes to know well his patients and their families.

The work of the general practitioner is predominantly concerned with the more common and 'minor' illnesses.

Various studies quoted by the College of General Practitioners (1965) (Reports from General Practice No. 2, "Present State and Future Needs"), show that between one-half and two-thirds of his work falls into this category of minor severity. One role of the general practitioner, therefore, is to protect hospitals and other specialist services from such conditions as can be managed by the general practitioners and it is he who has the task of assessing his patients as to their need for hospital and specialist services. The general practitioner with good diagnostic facilities will probably refer only 5 to 10 per cent of all patients seen to a specialist.

Fig. 9 illustrates the flow of care between the general practitioner and specialist services in the UK.

ADMINISTRATIVE STRUCTURE

The general medical service is a separate administrative unit in the NHS.

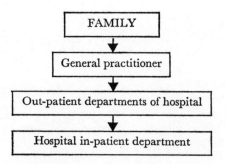

Fig. 9. Flow of care in the UK – to show place of GP.

The administrative units are the *Executive Councils*, which are responsible to the Department of Health. There are 134 Executive Councils in England and Wales, and they are independent and separate from the hospital and public health services with no corresponding territorial boundaries between the three branches.

The Executive Councils are concerned with paying the physician, keeping lists of patients registered with each general practitioner, acting as the centre to which any complaints from patients or doctors may be made, and with translating and implementing any decisions relating to general practice taken by Parliament and the Department of Health. They are responsible also for administering the dental, ophthalmic and pharmaceutical services.

The Executive Councils have not been involved in planning general medical services, nor in building medical premises, nor in carrying out any operational or other studies. They have no control or directive powers in planning and organising the general medical services in their areas. This is left to the physicians who remain quite independent in this respect.

THE WORK

The *nature of the morbidity pattern* of work in general practice in the UK is shown in Table 14.

Preventive work varies according to the views of the physi-

TABLE 14

Annual prevalence per 1,000 at risk of expected
morbidity in UK general practice

	Rates per 1,000 at risk
Minor illness	
Upper respiratory infections	200
Common digestive disorders	120
Skin disorders	120
Minor emotional problems	100
Acute otitis media	20
'Acute back'	20
Acute urinary infections	20
Migraine	12
Major illness	
Acute bronchitis and pneumonia	20
Coronary heart disease	6 (new cases 3)
Severe depression	5
All cancers (new cases)	2–3
Acute appendicitis	2
Chronic illness	
Chronic rheumatism	40
Chronic emotional illness	24
Chronic bronchitis	20
Anaemia	16
Hypertension	10
Asthma	10
Peptic Ulcers	10
'Strokes'	6
Diabetes	4
Epilepsy	4
Pulmonary (TB) (all cases)	1

(Source: Fry, J. *Profiles of Disease*, London (1966).)

cian and does not follow any standard pattern. If, as many
do, the physician carries out his own child welfare work,
then the proportion of such work will account for some 5
per cent of all his work. 'Routine medical check-ups' for
adults are not yet a part of British medical care.

The *population* for which the general practitioner is responsible is approximately 2,500 persons.

The *volume of work* involved in providing care for this population is shown in Tables 15 and 16.

Most of the work takes place in the consulting room but an appreciable number of home visits are made each day. The work is carried out quickly and the physician spends only 6–7 minutes on each of the 30–35 consultations in his office. He visits 10–12 patients in their homes, and each visit may only average 17 minutes, including travel. Night calls are few, perhaps only one or two every two or three weeks.

TABLE 15

Work pattern of British GPs

	Office consultations	Home visits	Hospital visits*	Total items of work	Time spent (hours)
A week	175	60	nil	235	35–45
A day	35	12	nil	47	7–9
Per cent	75%	25%	nil	—	—

* Most general practitioners do not visit their patients in hospital.
(Source: College of General Practitioners (1965). Reports from General Practice No. 2, "Present State and Future Needs".)

ACCESS AND AVAILABILITY

There are no problems relating to access or accessibility in first-contact care in the UK. In general outlying rural areas do not suffer from a deficiency of medical services, but it is becoming more difficult to recruit general practitioners into working in the less attractive industrial areas.

With complete freedom of choice of doctor and patient it is technically easy for persons to change doctor if they so wish by registering with another doctor after undertaking the necessary administrative procedure, but such changes are infrequent. Less than 1 per cent, in fact, change their doctors because of dissatisfaction.

First Contact Care

The British general practitioner is the most independent physician in the NHS. He may organise his work as he wishes, provide his own premises and engage his own staff and equip himself.

A major trend in general practice in the UK in recent years has been the move away from single-handed, practice to partnerships and group practice, and the single-handed general practitioner now represents less than 20 per cent of all physicians in general practice. The majority now prefer to work in small partnerships of 2, 3 or 4 physicians, working where possible from a single central premises.

Such group practice is encouraged by the NHS and each physician in a group of 3 or more working from central premises receives extra remuneration as an incentive.

There is also a move towards basing groups in community health centres. A health centre, of which there are now more than 60 (and a further 300 are planned within the next decade) enables up to 10–20 physicians to work together with paramedical auxiliaries, such as public health nurses, from one building to serve populations of 25,000–50,000 persons.

PLACE OF WORK

The premises from which the general practitioner in the UK works tends to be a private house adapted to medical needs. The College of General Practitioners (Report from General Practice No. 2 1965) reports tha': many of the present premises are old and facilities poor. New purpose-built premises are being built by physicians for themselves, with government aid, or by local authorities, but they represent as yet, no more than one-fifth of all general practices.

FACILITIES

Modern diagnostic facilities such as radiology and pathological services are not provided by the general practitioners themselves and such facilities are usually available at the local hospital. General practitioners can refer their patients directly to the laboratory or for radiology, with the investigations being carried out on their instructions and the reports sent to the physician.

The investigations requested by the general practitioner fall within the 'simple' range and experience has shown that these do not add a significant burden to the work of the laboratory or radiology departments at the local hospital.

Access to hospital beds for general practitioners is unusual, and although there are some hospitals that provide beds in which general practitioners can treat their own patients, these are exceptional.

General practitioners can work in hospital departments as 'Clinical Assistants' under the direction of the specialist in charge.

HEALTH TEAM

In the UK there have been moves towards integration, through the development of 'health teams' in the community, thus bridging the communication gaps between the hospital and community services.

The physician can no longer work alone to provide the care required and expected at first-contact level, for if he is to devote his time to conditions, problems and situations requiring the medical skills for which he has been trained he must be able to delegate some of his present tasks to paramedical colleagues.

There are now many 'health teams' in the UK working together. Comprising general practitioners, nurses, health visitors (public health nurses trained to deal with social problems, health education and preventive care), medical secretaries and more specialised ancillaries such as mental welfare officers, these 'health teams' have found that by working together they can provide care for larger populations than when working alone.

A typical composition of a health team serving a population of 10,000 would be as follows:

TABLE 16
First-contact health team in the UK for 10,000 persons

Physicians (general practitioners)	3
Nurses	2
Health visitor (medical social worker)	1
Medical secretaries	4
Midwife	1
Mental welfare officer	$\frac{1}{2}$ (attached to 2 units)

This health team which comprises employees of local authorities as well as those employed by the physician, provides medical, social and preventive care required at the first-contact level. This care includes antenatal supervision, child welfare, clinical medical management, health education and pre-symptomatic screening.

It also assists with the many and various social, personal and family problems that occur within its community. In managing these it refers some to other social agencies and skilled personnel. Thus, the mental welfare officer is brought in to help in the care of the more complex emotional problems in the community, whereas the 'Home Help' services are called in to help in domestic work for the sick, disabled and elderly on a temporary or permanent basis. Special services are available also for the blind, the deaf, the handicapped and for special social situations such as 'problem families'.

EDUCATION AND TRAINING

Some of the current problems of general practice in the UK have arisen from deficiencies of education in community health at the undergraduate level and from an ineffective system of postgraduate vocational training.

REWARDS AND INCENTIVES

General practitioners working in the NHS are paid by a combination of annual capitation fees for each registered person plus a variety of extras based on incentives towards agreed policies. Thus they receive extra remuneration for each elderly person (over 65); for night calls; for persons who stay only temporarily in their area; for maternity care; for preventive measures such as immunisations and cervical cytology. They also receive some reimbursement for the salaries of secretaries and nurses that they employ and for rates and rent spent on their premises.

Extra payments are made for seniority, for postgraduate education courses attended, for an approved vocational training, for working in groups of 3 or more physicians from central premises, and for working in areas that are 'under-doctored'.

Approximately 3 out of 4 of all UK citizens consult their general practitioners once or more each year. The mean numbers of consultation are between 3 and 4 per person each year.

Utilisation of available resources is also subject to considerable variations, as for example, in the use of diagnostic facilities, rates of referral to specialists and in-patient admissions by an individual physician (College of General Practitioners, 1965, Report from General Practice No. 2, "Present State and Future Needs").

Direct Comparisons of First-Contact Care

THE PLACE OF THE DOCTOR-OF-FIRST-CONTACT
(PRIMARY PHYSICIAN)

In the three systems the doctor-of-first-contact has similar roles to play and his work in each of the three countries has inevitably certain common features.

He provides the *first point of medical contact* for the patient. As such he acts as an assessor of his patient's needs and having made his assessment he next has to decide whether he can manage the problem or whether referral to more specialised services is required.

The doctor-of-first-contact tends to work in a fairly *static community* and to provide care for a relatively *small population*. Except in the situation in the USA where young physicians in hospital emergency rooms provide first-contact care for medical indigents, primary physicians in the USSR the USA and the UK appear to be responsible for similar sized populations, namely, 2,500 to 4,000, of whom 500 to 1,000 will be children under 15 years.

Working in a static and small population of this size, the primary physician has opportunities to provide *long-term and continuing care* for his patients. These opportunities appear more easily achieved in the USSR and the UK than in the USA since in their systems of care frequent changes of physician are discouraged.

The patterns of work facing these physicians are similar. The *morbidity spectrum* is that which occurs in populations of

85

2,500 to 4,000 persons with similar social and economic standards.

In each nation the primary physician is faced with more than managing the purely clinical problems. Personal and family situations arise and must be managed, with difficulties relating to local social problems influencing care, whilst the challenges of early diagnosis and prevention have also to be faced.

Access to the primary physician is free and unobstructed in the USSR and the UK. Within these systems the patient has his or her regular physician whom he or she can contact in times of need. In the USSR the local or *uchastok* physician, or her deputy, is available constantly at the local polyclinic, and in the UK patients are registered with a general practitioner who by contract has to be available, or provide a deputy, at all times.

In the USA group practices or other pre-paid insurance schemes are under contract to provide direct access for the patient. Elsewhere the system of fees-for-services creates barriers for some. The tradition of one patient one doctor is not customary in the USA so there is no strong bond whereby the physician feels bound to be available and accessible to his patients at all times.

The principle of *free choice of physician* differs in the three nations.

In the USSR there is no free choice. With the *uchastok* principle all persons living in a prescribed neighbourhood are allocated to the physician responsible for that geographical zone.

In the UK there is free choice in theory. The patient can, under the NHS, apply to any general practitioner to be accepted as his patient. In practice, however, the choice is inevitably limited to those general practitioners within the immediate locality and the tendency is for physicians to limit their practices within easy travel distances and not to accept patients living too far away. In urban regions, where 80 per cent of the UK live, the physician will often not accept persons living more than $\frac{1}{2}$–1 mile away.

In the USA there is complete free choice, but this freedom is bound by financial barriers, namely, ability to pay the fees. It is restricted also by geography, and in many outlying areas not only is there no free choice, but there is no choice at all because there are no physicians in practice for many miles. Over-emphasis on free choice sometimes leads to frequent changes of physician with ensuing lack of continuity, duplicity and confusion in care.

The place of the first-contact physician in the *flow of medical care* differs in the three systems.

Fig. 10 illustrates some of these differences. In the UK the general practitioner is the main portal of entry into the NHS.

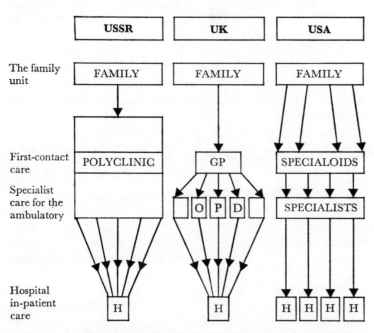

Fig. 10. A comparison of the flow of medical care in the USSR, UK and USA.

In the USSR it is the *uchastok* physicians in the local polyclinic who are the first medical contacts, but there are different primary physicians for children, for the parents, and for persons suffering from certain diseases. In the USA a family group often has a multiplicity of primary physicians, few of whom know that others are caring for other members of the family.

First Contact Care

In the UK the generalist family doctor has been perpe-tuated through the NHS. In the USSR all physicians, including the first-contact physicians are recognised as 'specialists'. In the USA the trend is towards a specialist primary physician, but at present there is a grand mixture of various types of physicians carrying out the work.

What is a 'specialist'? Classification is necessary if his place in first-contact care is to be understood. The usual connotation of medical specialist is that he is a physician who practises in a restricted clinical or paraclinical field and who, because of such restrictions, deals with the more complex and obscure conditions. He is recognised as a specialist by his colleagues, and they refer patients to him for his expert advice and opinions, usually such recognition only follows a long and accepted course of training followed by an examination and certification.

Is the field of first-contact medical care a speciality and can a physician specialise in it?

Undoubtedly special skills, knowledge and training are necessary and for this reason it can be recognised as a speciality. Whether within this specialty it is possible to subdivide the work into paediatrics and adult medicine and other recognised sub-groups is however question-able.

For example the primary paediatrician in this field will spend one-third of his time in routine well-child care, a quarter of his time in caring for minor upper respiratory infection and much of the rest of his time with other minor and self-limiting childhood ailments. He will encounter only rarely the more severe and more difficult clinical problems that form the normal casework of a paediatrician who works in hospital. There must, therefore be a distinction between the specialoid first-contact (or primary) paediatri-cian and the paediatric specialist who is recognised as a consultant.

Similar reasoning must apply to other specialities such as internal medicine, obstetrics and gynaecology.

Does first-contact medical care require generalists or specialoids?

All three systems provide good service for most of their population. It is not possible to state that any is best, but it is important to try and evaluate through further comparative studies what resources are required in the various systems to achieve comparable end results.

The advantages of a generalist first-contact physician are that he is able to function as a family doctor and is able to fit into a community health team with relative ease.

However, the advantages of a specialoid in this field are that he (or she) is able to concentrate more definitively on the problems relating to a special group of the population, albeit dealing with the common and less serious conditions. It is easier for such a physician to undergo a course of training and easier for him to work in a hospital-orientated system, as in the USA, where primary physicians have ready access to hospitals.

TRAINING, STATUS, INCENTIVES AND CAREER STRUCTURE

Vocational Training

In the USSR many newly qualified medical graduates are directed into first-contact medical care as part of their three-year post-qualification period during which they may be directed into any appointment anywhere in the Soviet Republic. This direction of labour is accepted by the young physician as the responsibility of a Soviet citizen.

Training is of an in-service nature. The junior physician is attached to a polyclinic to work under the supervision of more senior colleagues. In addition there are set periods for postgraduate studies. Thus, for three months each year the more junior staff of polyclinics exchange their work with their colleagues in local hospitals in order to maintain their experience in hospital care and developments.

Every three years all physicians in the USSR are required to attend postgraduate courses in their speciality, and this applies to local *uchastok* physicians as well as to others.

In the USA the nature of the vocational training is left to the individual physician, but is guided by the new speciality in family medicine and general practice. The training undertaken is entirely hospital based and orientated, and comprises a series of hospital appointments considered by the young physician to be of possible value in his future career.

Many carry out a longer hospital training in a specific subject in order to achieve Board Certification in internal medicine or paediatrics or some other speciality. Board certified primary physicians find it easier to be accepted as a specialist in their work and to be accepted for full privileges at the local hospitals.

In the UK vocational training for general practice has been based on an apprenticeship 'trainee assistant' scheme, following one or more years of general hospital work. Under this scheme young physicians are attached to recognised senior practitioners who act as their tutors for a year or more. In the future, it is likely that more organised training over 3–4 years will lead to registration as a 'specialist', according to the Royal Commission on Medical Education Report in 1968.

Status

The status of the doctor-of-first-contact is not high in any of the systems.

Largely neglected as a branch of medical care worthy of special teaching in undergraduate medical schools, most medical students qualify with the impression that to be a doctor-of-first-contact no special skills or training are required.

In the USA and the UK there has been a steady and notable withdrawal of physicians from this field and relative shortages of such physicians are occurring in socially unattractive localities.

In the USSR no such problems arise because of the powers of the State in the direction of physicians. Another factor is that work in this field is particularly satisfying and convenient for women, who account for 4 out of 5 of all local physicians.

Incentives and Rewards

The systems of remuneration are quite different.

In the USSR all physicians are paid by salary that is

related to experience, seniority and merit, as determined by higher qualifications and achievements.

In the USA fees-for-services are the standard method of remuneration. The scales of fees are determined by individual practitioners with guidance from their professional organisations.

In the UK the system of remuneration is through a combination of annual capitation fees and extras from the State for all those patients registered with the general practitioner.

Whatever the reasons, primary physicians in the USSR and the USA seem happier and more satisfied with their professional lives than do their colleagues in the UK.

Career Structure

Work in the first-contact field is recognised in the USSR as a stepping stone to more specialised branches of medicine. In fact, priority is often given in the selection of candidates for specialist training and appointments to those who have spent time as local *uchastok* physicians.

For those who remain in this branch there is a recognised career structure with progression through seniority, ability and merit.

In the USA a flexible attitude exists for interchange between the first-contact and the more specialised fields of medical care.

In the UK such movement in and out of the various levels of specialisation in the medical profession is exceptional. The NHS with its rigid subdivisions of medical care into general practice, hospital work and public health service, has made it almost impossible for physicians, once established in one of the three branches, to move into another.

THE WORK AND UTILISATION OF SERVICES

The work and the nature of the morbidity dealt with by the physician-of-first-contact is everywhere similar. Differences in detail that do exist such as the proportions and numbers of persons suffering from emotional problems, obesity, hypertension, coronary heart disease or chronic chest ailments are often related to local medical nomenclature and to special prevailing social and environmental factors. The important fact is that everywhere the first-contact physician deals primarily with the less serious and more common ailments of a small, static and defined community.

Organisation of work depends on the system and local conditions. Most patients are seen by the physician in his consulting rooms.

In the USSR and the UK home visiting still represents a considerable proportion of the work, but in the USA home visiting has been reduced drastically.

Because physicians in the USA have access to hospitals, visits to patients under their care in hospital beds account for an appreciable proportion of their work. (Table 17.)

TABLE 17
Work loads of doctors-of-first-contact

	USSR	USA		UK
UTILISATION RATES (Annual attendances per patient to doctor-of-first-contact)	3–6 (excluding dental vists and attendances to polyclinic specialists)	4–5		3–5
VOLUME OF WORK (Doctor-patient contacts in one week)		*Internist*	*'GP'*	
Office consultations	85	55	100	175
Home visits	35	5	15	60
Hospital visits	—	25	50	—
TOTAL	129	85	165	235
TIME PER PATIENT				
Office consultation	12 min.	25 min.		6–7 min.
Home visit	30 min.	30 min.		16–18 min.
PHYSICIAN'S WORKING WEEK (Time spent in contact with patients)	35 hours	35–40 hours		35–45 hours

(Sources: USSR: Popov, G.A. (1967), personal communication. USA: Kroeger, H.H., *et al.* (1965), and Eimerl, T.S. (1967). UK: College of General Practitioners (1965).)

The volume of work and the utilisation rates of equivalent physicians is shown in Table 17.

The utilisation rates for the USSR normally quoted include attendances for dental treatment and referrals to specialists.

Attendances for dental care and specialist referrals are excluded from data quoted from the USA and the UK. If these attendances are also exluded from the USSR rates then the rates of utilisation of all three countries become remarkably similar.

The *volume of work* carried out by the average primary physician, however, differs appreciably.

The British general practitioner sees almost twice as many patients in the same working week as do his colleagues in the USSR and the USA. As a consequence he spends much less time on each consultation and he must by inference do less at each contact for his patient.

Whether the end results are any different in terms of the health of the community, it is however impossible to determine.

STRUCTURE, ADMINISTRATION AND PLACE OF WORK

Administration

First-contact care in the USSR is an integral part of medical care. Neighbourhood *uchastok* physicians fit easily and recognisably into the activities of the polyclinic and the polyclinics are related closely with the District hospital and the public health (sanepid) service.

The administration of each polyclinic is under the direction of the chief physician who in turn is responsible to the chief physician of the District the administrative head of all the medical care services in his district, including polyclinics.

The situation is different in the USA. Independent primary physicians are free to practise where they please and there is no system of overall planning and administration or control.

In the UK there is a mixture of professional independence coupled with administrative controls by the local Executive Councils of the NHS. The physician is free to apply to practise where he wishes but he must have the approval of the Executive Council. This is granted automatically in areas where there is not already an excessive number of physicians. Private practice can be carried out anywhere and is free of any restrictions.

Whilst the Executive Councils are concerned to ensure that the public can receive organised medical care, physicians are quite free and independent to organise their day-to-day work according to their wishes and beliefs.

Place of Work

Similar trends are notable in all countries with the centralisation of facilities and grouping of physicians occuring in the USSR, the USA and the UK.

The polyclinics of the USSR are central medical centres serving communities up to 50,000 and providing a base for up to 150 physicians – both specialists and primary physicians.

Whilst the majority of the primary physicians, in the USA still work alone from their own offices there has nevertheless been a trend towards group practice. Group practices may comprise from 3 to 100 physicians working from central premises with good facilities for general and special care and investigations.

Partnerships of 2, 3 or 4 general practitioners have been common in the UK for many years, even before the NHS. Since 1948 this trend has increased and now less than 1 in 5 of British general practitioners work alone.

These groups and partnerships still tend to be small and few comprise more than 5 physicians (less than 10 per cent of all practices are groups of more than 5).

The pattern in the UK is for groups of general practitioners to work from their own adapted premises which are small and have few modern diagnostic and therapeutic facilities.

The Health Team

The modern physician must work in close association with his paramedical colleagues and this applies to the field of first-contact care as elsewhere.

The USSR has had a strong force of middle-grade workers for many generations. The 'feldshers' still occupy important and essential roles in rural areas, where they provide the points of medical first contact. In addition to their work with minor clinical matters their tasks range across health education, public health administration, preventive care and social rehabilitation. They work closely with, and are supervised by, the local physician.

Each local physician has a trained nurse working with him and these nurses combine general office administration with the nursing duties required in the polyclinics and on home visits.

The work of nurse and physician is often shared, but there are considerable overlaps and sometimes a notable lack of delegation from physician to nurse.

In the USA with the system of private medical care, where the patients pay for the physicians' services, there have been few opportunities and fewer incentives for bringing middle-grade nurse-social workers into any health team. Patients who pay the physician are reluctant to be cared for by his paramedical employees.

With impending shortages of physicians the climate in the USA is ready for developing the concept of a community health team, and experiments in certain centres, usually in less affluent regions amongst medical indigents, using paramedical workers to perform some of the physicians' traditional tasks, are now being conducted.

The American health team at present tends to comprise nurses and medical secretaries employed privately by the physician. Their roles are to assist the physician to carry out his work as speedily and as efficiently as possible in his office and not to undertake any delegated roles in the actual care of the patients.

The UK has, as the USSR had, a well-recognised place for middle-grade medical workers for almost the last century, the health visitors.

These public health nurses were originally created to meet the deficiencies in the care of young children of mothers who could not afford to take them to a physician. In order that they did not compete with the medical work of physicians, health visitors are restricted from any therapeutic tasks and are involved in preventive and educational work only.

Times have changed and so have the roles of these highly trained workers, who undergo a full nursing, midwifery, social, preventive and health educational course lasting five or more years.

Many health visitors, who are employed by local public health authorities, are now attached to general practices to work with general practitioners in providing more comprehensive and co-operative care.

Their work in general practice now extends beyond child welfare to antenatal care, support of problem families, mental disorders, the handicapped, the elderly and the chronic sick and various other types of social pathology.

Other members of the general practice health team in the UK are nurses, who may be employed by the physicians or delegated to them by local authorities. Medical secretaries and more specialised social workers such as mental welfare officers are often members of the staff, part or full-time in the larger groups.

An increasing proportion of previously considered physician-type work is now being delegated to these other members of the health team who work under the supervision and direction of the physician.

Associations with the Hospital

Major differences exist in the systems of hospital association in all three countries.

In the USA general access to hospital beds and other facilities is accepted as part of the rights of most primary physicians. These physicians are able to treat their own patients, charging fees for the various ailments treated in hospital.

In the USSR and the UK access to hospital beds for primary physicians is exceptional and occurs only in rural areas and in small hospitals. In both nations, however, many hospitals provide direct diagnostic facilities for local physicians.

A Personal Evaluation

The subject of access to hospital beds by primary physicians must raise some questions that are of considerable importance to the evaluation of medical care in any community.

1. *The competence of the Physician and the Quality of Care*

In view of the limited opportunities for a primary physician to develop any wide experience in the less common and more complex conditions, how competent is he to undertake full responsibility for his patients with hospital-type conditions? Recalling that in a population of 2,500 persons it can be expected that 5 or fewer cases of appendicitis will occur each year; some 10 patients will sustain acute chest infections and respiratory failure; 5–10 patients will have acute myocardial infarcts; and fewer than 5 women suffer obstetric complications, how much continuing experience does a physician need to remain safe and competent? If he is allowed such responsibilities then undoubtedly the quality of care received by the patients will be less expert than that provided by teams of specialists.

2. *The Financial Incentives*

If the physician works in hospital then he must be remunerated. However, it is important that the financial incentives should not be so great as to encourage him to undertake work there, on behalf of his patients, for which he is not qualified.

3. *The Benefits to Physician and Patient*

The benefits of an association between primary physician and hospital are appreciable to physician, hospital and patient. For the physician, the benefits are those of professional association with colleagues and the growing points of medicine. This leads to a continuing educational process which must ultimately be of benefit to the patient. For the hospital, association with the primary physician creates a link with the community and provides extra medical staff. For the patient, care in hospital from a known physician who understands the patient's personal problems makes for greater confidence and comfort.

4. *The Problems of the Hospital*

Open access of beds to local physicians creates problems over the numbers of staff concerned in that building, in patient treatment. In the USA where such access exists, there are hospitals of 200–300 beds that boast a medical staff of over 800 physicians.

5. *The Possible Alternatives*

A continuing association between the practising doctors-of-first-contact and local hospitals is a feature of good medical care, for it is particularly useful both as a continuing educational exercise for the physician and to allow the patient in hospital to be cared for by his own physician.

In the USA and the USSR the principle of association is accepted and applied. In the USA there is full access with full responsibilities in many areas. In the USSR the local physicians work for three months of each year in hospital as a result of an exchange with hospital physicians. In the UK there are at present tenuous associations and minimal access to beds. There seem therefore to be three possible alternatives:

(*a*) For primary physicians to have full access and responsibility for undertaking hospital care for their patients and to leave decisions as to his own competence to the physician.

(*b*) For primary physicians to have restricted facilities. These restrictions to apply to the care of certain agreed and recognised conditions. Thus most surgical procedures would be excluded.

(*c*) For primary physicians to work in hospitals as members of teams or units, e.g. attached to a paediatric or medical unit, or as a member of the psychiatric or obstetric team and as such be under the direction of a specialist.

Some Implications of the Study of the Systems in the Three Countries

1. *Do we still need a doctor-of-first-contact?*

The answer to this justifiable question must be – 'YES'.

Without such a method of care both the patient and the system of medical care will suffer. The patient needs a primary physician who is recognisable and whose roles are clearly understood. He must be someone to whom the patient has direct access in times of medical need and who will be able to guide his patients safely through the medical jungle with its modern snares and hazards. Patients all over the world seek such a physician who is able also to provide personal long-term and continuing care and who at the same time is familiar with the family and its background.

Any system of medical care must have a sound and reliable service of first-contact care. There has to be at the first level of medical care, where the more common and less complex disorders of the community may be managed without referral to the more expensive and highly expert hospitals, a primary physician.

Primary physicians have the important function of serving as a protective screen around the hospitals.

Where there are no doctors-of-first contact in the community then the hospital becomes the point of first contact, e.g. the hospital emergency rooms of some hospitals in the USA provide care for medical indigents, and becomes involved in caring for conditions which do not necessarily require the facilities of a modern hospital.

2. *If we do need a primary physician, what place should he occupy?*

A well-defined place with accepted roles and functions must be established if this branch of medical care is to be of high quality, satisfying to the physician and appreciated by the patient. The primary physician's chief responsibilities must be with the care of the ordinary and common medical and social problems that occur in our communities. He must be prepared to refer the more extraordinary and more difficult and complex problems to specialists. His place in any system must be accepted as important and his work as worth while, with its own special expertise and skills, that have to be taught and learnt.

His role will be to act as the doctor-of-first-contact to whom patients have direct access; to provide personal and continuing care to his patients who form a relatively small and static community; and to become expert in the diagnosis, assessment and management of the conditions that commonly occur in such a community.

The tools that he requires are many.

The physician must receive specific education and training for the work that he will undertake, similar in duration and depth to that of other specialities (see *Royal Commission on Medical Education 1963–1968*, HMSO, London, 1968).

Whether he be a generalist or a specialoid will depend on local beliefs and attitudes, but perhaps in the end it makes little difference if either type is able to meet the challenge of his defined roles. Professional facilities must include purpose-built premises, access to modern diagnostic and therapeutic tools and equipment and there must be suitably trained staff with whom he can work and to whom he may delegate and refer cases. Furthermore close and integral association with hospitals and other services is essential if high quality is to be maintained.

3. *A Basic Blueprint*

Taking the 'best' out of the three systems, the following may serve as a blueprint for the future.

(*a*) The first-contact branch of the medical system must be recognised as a distinct unit. It must have its own recognisable career structure with an education and training programme that is recognised as being up to the standard of other specialities. The education must commence in the medical schools and the training must be specific and vocational in character and with suitable measures of quality, through examinations and other periodic assessments.

Planned teaching should be organised by special departments concerned with this field as a part of community medical care. Such departments would inevitably be concerned with research as well as teaching.

The status of this branch must be recognised by the rest of the profession, but such a status cannot be achieved unless its roles and functions are understood and a high quality of care seen to be carried out. Such appreciation and understanding require that all future physicians receive education on this subject.

(*b*) Medical care should be planned on districts. District plans should be drawn up in close cooperation with those who work in that district. Local physicians and their paramedical colleagues should have the continuing opportunities to prepare five- or ten-year plans for their own district taking into account known and established problems, defects and needs.

(*c*) An integrated system combining primary care with the local hospital and public health services is rational, necessary and obviously possible, as demonstrated in the USSR where all the medical services of an area are integrated under the direction of a single person, the chief physician of the District.

(*d*) First-contact services must be centralised into larger units from which health teams comprising physicians, nurses and other paramedical colleagues can provide care in a co-operative fashion. Each health team should have its own known population, whether this be geographical as in the USSR *uchastok* principle or through free-choice registration as in the UK is probably unimportant. What is important is that the population at risk is known in order that preventive and continuing care may be planned and organised.

(*e*) Association with hospitals is important for the primary physician. Its importance probably lies more in continuing education of the physician than the quality of the service that he can give to his patients for their hospital-type diseases.

Chapter 5
Specialist Ambulatory Care

Between first-contact care and the hospital, there is a need for specialist care for patients who are ambulatory.

Such specialists may function as consultant clinicians, available for advice and guidance to other physicians, or serve as experts specially skilled in diagnostic or therapeutic procedures and who may be called in to act as 'technicians' to perform specific tasks.

The specialist, is one who is recognised as such by both public and profession and who has undergone a recognised postgraduate training usually followed by a certifying examination.

The population from which his patients come is much larger than that of a primary physician. Thus in the UK one general surgeon may be required for a population of 50–75,000, and a neurologist for a population up to 500,000 in contrast to 2,500 persons cared for by a general practitioner.

Whilst in some systems of medical care patients may have direct access to specialists, referral (of patients) from other physicians is the hall-mark of a consultant specialist and as a consultant the clinical specialist does not often provide long-term and continuing care. He will require access to expensive and complex diagnostic and therapeutic facilities.

The Specialist in the USSR

The specialist ambulatory services in Soviet Russia are based on the polyclinic, which is the centre of specialised medical care for the community outside the hospital, and therefore represents the core of the system of out-patient care.

In many respects it combines, and acts as, the focal point for many services that would be otherwise poorly related. It also cuts across and demolishes many intra-professional barriers.

The polyclinic houses various clinical and paraclinical specialists to care for ambulatory patients, and they may visit the homes of those patients who are unable to make the journey.

These specialists represent the second level in the dynamic flow of medical care in the USSR (Fig. 11) between the primary 'uchastok' physicians and those who work in hospitals.

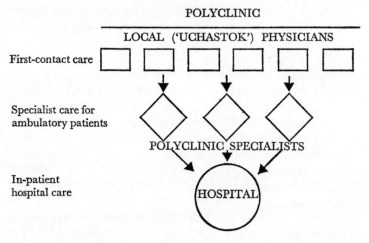

Fig. 11. Place of the polyclinic in medical care in the USSR.

The polyclinic specialist receives a recognised training and passes appropriate examinations in his speciality. In the polyclinic he serves as an out-patient specialist, responsible only for ambulatory patients. In the urban polyclinics they do not usually hold simultaneous hospital appointments, and although at times they return to hospital work for short periods or further postgraduate education, in practice when a patient is admitted to hospital he is cared for by a different set of specialists who work only in hospital. In rural areas the situation differs as the populations are smaller and the polyclinic and local hospital are often combined into a single unit with common staff.

Therefore the polyclinic specialist does not follow his patients into hopital. He is a specialist only in those conditions that he is able to manage on an ambulatory basis, and only for those patients in his speciality that occur in a population of 10,000–50,000 served by the polyclinic.

In addition to the medical and clinical work carried out, the polyclinic also serves as the local centre for many special paramedical social services. 'Feldshers' attached to the polyclinic act as general social workers and in particular fields such as occupational medicine, tuberculosis, maternity and child welfare and mental illness.

There are good links with the local public health service, where other social and public facilities are based. Since this service is responsible for a larger population than that of a single polyclinic, each public health area includes a number of polyclinics, but their physicians and other public health workers are often attached to the local polyclinics.

Links with the District hospital are of a formal nature. Communications tend to be by correspondence rather than through personal contact, because of the division and distinction between the two sets of staff.

There are exceptions to this division and certain hospital specialists with particular experience may conduct consulting sessions in some polyclinics, but this is not customary.

A major role of the polyclinic is participation in the 'dispenserisation scheme' of preventive screening and follow-up. This work involves the specialists as well as the local physicians.

There is real public involvement and representation in the work of each polyclinic, and there are elected representatives from the local community on the Management Board, although the actual administration is the responsibility of the Chief Physician of the polyclinic.

Many lay members of the public who have undergone some simple and basic health training help in the work of the polyclinic through assistance with activities such as health education, follow-up attendances and in general organisation of clinics. This work is done voluntarily and freely without any pay or other financial rewards.

GENERAL POLICIES AND TYPES OF POLYCLINICS

The siting and placing of polyclinics is part of the overall plan of medical care. The District Health Department decides on the siting of polyclinics in accordance with territorial and occupational divisions.

A compromise has to be reached between the benefits of centralising medical facilities and ensuring reasonable access to the public and thus different problems exist in rural and urban areas.

In rural areas with dispersed populations of from 2,000 to 10,000, the polyclinic is combined with a small local hospital and is related closely with outlying 'feldsher–midwife' posts.

In urban areas polyclinics are planned to serve 30–50,000 persons but with the development of large housing projects, with high-rise buildings some decentralisation is occurring and polyclinics are setting up satellite units in large blocks of flats, where local physicians and specialists can see patients.

Some of the new polyclinics are being sited within the grounds of District hospitals to improve liaison, but since there may be between three and six polyclinics in each District hospital area only one polyclinic can have the benefits of such closer geographical relations.

TYPES OF POLYCLINICS

The organisation and planning of the polyclinic services is a major task of the Regional Health Department.

In Moscow, which is recognised as a Region, there are some 600 polyclinics for its $6\frac{1}{2}$ million people. These include 164 adult polyclinics, 130 children's polyclinics, 63 industrial polyclinics, 121 women's consultation clinics and 21 dental polyclinics. There are in addition many (over 500) dispensaries (special polyclinics combined with in-patient facilities) for tuberculosis, neoplasms, skin and venereal diseases and mental illnesses.

Adult Care

In urban areas the adult polyclinic is a separate one, from that which caters for children, and it provides services only for those over the age of 15. The populations cared for by such a polyclinic range from 20,000 to 50,000.

Specialist Ambulatory Care

All urban polyclinics are built and organised on a common pattern and one I visited in Moscow is typical.

Situated in an old industrial area of Moscow it provides out-patient care for 41,000 persons, and purpose built in 1959 it has four floors and is constructed in traditional style from yellow brick.

It has a staff of 90 physicians, 133 paramedical workers, 20 clerical assistants and 15 cleaners.

Physicians

Local (*uchastok*) physicians	20
Specialist therapists (physicians)	10
Surgeons (minor surgery only)	5
ENT specialists	2
Urologist	1
Gynaecologist (diagnostic work only)	1
Pathologists	5
Radiologists	3
Infectious diseases	1
Ophthalmologists	3
Neuropathologists (psychiatrists)	5
Dental surgeons	13
Others (including physical medicine, rheumatology, etc.)	21
	90

Nurses	118
Feldshers	15
Clerks, etc.	20
Cleaners	15

It is open from 8 a.m. to 8 p.m., and in addition has two emergency units on call during the whole twenty-four hours and there is an emergency room for minor trauma.

The daily work load is between 1,000 and 1,500 consultations each day, and between 8 p.m. and 8 a.m. there are approximately 20–25 evening and night visits.

In addition to the residential population the polyclinic is responsible for two local factories, each with an industrial health unit and each staffed by the polyclinic with a physician and four feldshers.

Child Care

Wherever possible the children's polyclinic is separate from
that for adults and they care for a child population of between
10,000 and 15,000. They are not intended to care for the sick
child, and the child who is sick and feverish will be visited in
its home. At Poltava, for example, which is a city of 185,000
in the Ukraine, the polyclinic was in a children's hospital of
125 beds (serving 38,000 children).

There were 42 physicians and 142 nurses working here
and 14 of these physicians were local '*uchastok*' paediatricians
each caring for 800 children, and the other 28 staff being
specialists.

In Moscow one of the children's polyclinics, responsible for
the care of 15,000 children in an area of three-mile radius,
looked after: 8 schools, 5 nurseries, 5 kindergartens and 14
nurseries.

This polyclinic truly served as the local medical centre for
children, and about 750 attendances were made to the polyclinic daily.

The staff consisted of:

Physicians

Local (*uchastok*) paediatricians	27
School doctors	8

Specialists

ENT	2
Psychiatrist	1
General surgeon	1
Orthopaedic surgeon	1
'Rheumatic fever' specialist	1
Dermatologist	1
Tuberculosis (visiting)	1
Endocrinologist	1
Nephrologist	1
Physiotherapist	1
Physical culture	1
Dental surgeon	1
Ophthalmologist	1
Immunologist	1
Radiologist	1
Pathologist	1

Nurses

Local (*uchastok*) nurses	22
'Feldshers' at schools	8
General nurses	59

The range of specialisation at this polyclinic must be considered as very generous when it is realised that a population of only 15,000 children is being cared for and that these specialists do not have hospital appointments.

The Women's Clinic

These are polyclinics that provide specialist care for gynaecological and obstetric conditions, and they offer antenatal and postnatal care, with preventive services such as cervical cytology and routine examinations, with health education.

In addition they have an even greater social role for they also act as advisory centres for women, providing advice on marital problems, family planning and legal abortions.

One such Clinic in Moscow served a population of 160,000 (90,000 females), covering a radius of 5 miles, and was associated closely with a maternity hospital but the medical staffs were different.

The medical staff of the polyclinic comprised 28 physicians and 35 trained midwives – none of whom was responsible for the actual delivery which takes place in hospital

Dispensaries

The dispensary is a more specialised polyclinic caring for conditions such as tuberculosis, neoplasms, skin and venereal diseases, psychiatric conditions, eye disorders and others, and some dispensaries are part of a special hospital as was the TB dispensary I visited in Moscow.

This TB dispensary provided care for a population of 350,000, and included a unit with 150 beds, an out-patient department, a day centre for 25 persons, a sheltered workshop and diagnostic facilities.

The staff comprised 45 physicians and 110 nurses, involved in both in-patient and out-patient care.

Some 200–350 new cases of tuberculosis are dealt with each year (6–10 per 10,000) at the dispensary and approximately 1,200 active cases are under supervision at any time.

The Dental Clinic

In larger cities there are separate dental polyclinics that act as special referral centres for complex situations and which also provide routine dental care for the local population. In rural areas, as in the Ukraine, such polyclinics also organise mobile dental units that visit outlying areas for regular dental care of the population.

The Industrial Clinic (Medical Sanitary Unit)

At larger industrial establishments which employ 5,000 or more workers living close by, polyclinics have been set up to provide general and occupational care for the workers and their families and this clinic is part of a more extensive system of care for workers.

In addition to the polyclinic that provides the customary first-contact and specialist services, there may be also a hospital in the unit.

The occupational health work is organised on the *uchastok* (or neighbourhood) principle, and the industrial unit is divided into sub-units where each occupational physician is given the responsibility for the care of about 1,000 workers.

The tasks of this physician include specific preventive work with occupational diseases and industrial injuries, improvement of working conditions in his sub-unit, health screening, preventive immunisations and general health education.

Working with these specialist occupational physicians are specially trained 'feldshers' who have their own health posts in the establishment, who implement some of the preventive activities and also deal with minor medical problems.

A special and unique facility in industry is the 'prophylactorium.'

This is a special type of residential unit with up to 100 beds designed to provide preventive care for workers who are in danger of breaking down from physical and non-physical disorders. Their main feature is that they provide after-work accommodation, including sleeping facilities and offer opportunities for group therapy and individual care. Members of the families are invited to attend some of the group sessions.

Vulnerable individuals found to be suffering from conditions such as peptic ulcers, rheumatism, hypertension, cardiac lesions, chronic bronchitis, tuberculosis or emotional problems are recommended by the physicians for such treatment and they report to the 'prophylactorium' on completion of their work-shift. They are provided with meals and residential accommodation and in addition receive group therapy, rehabilitation and specific medical treatment which may include hydrotherapy and physiotherapy. During their period of care they are supervised by the physicians and nurses attached to the prophylactorium.

The patient attends on average regularly and daily (but not at week-ends) for a month and then for follow-up. The aims are to allow treatment, and especially preventive measures, to be carried out whilst the worker remains at his job.

Approximately one-half of the medical work of a polyclinic is carried out by the specialists and the other half by the local *uchastok* physicians.

The specialists' work in the polyclinic is thus somewhat restricted, and a surgeon's technical work will be confined to ambulatory surgery, including certain diagnostic procedures such as sigmoidoscopy, to minor surgery such as excision of cysts and minor trauma. Cases that require admission will not be dealt with by him, but by his colleagues in hospital.

Current trends in the USSR however are towards larger polyclinics with better facilities serving larger populations, of up to 50–60,000. It is also proposed that there will be more separate specialised polyclinics, but it must be noted that this will lead to even more dispersal of care of the individual patient.

The Specialist in the USA

There is no clearly defined sector of specialist ambulatory medical care in the USA, but a spectrum that ranges from the specialist acting as a doctor-of-first-contact to the super-specialist who sees patients only by referral for the most rare disorders.

The pattern of organisation of specialist ambulatory care depends on the locale and on social, economic and geographical factors, but three types of care can be recognised, namely the solo specialist in private practice, the group of specialists working together, and those working at a hospital out-patient service.

PRIVATE CARE BY INDIVIDUAL SPECIALISTS

Board certified specialists practise from their own consulting suites, often in purpose-built privately owned buildings, providing their own staff and making their own arrangements for diagnostic procedures. These they may carry out themselves or the patients may be referred to colleagues also in private practice, and for therapy which is often on a continuing basis requiring regular attendances and supervision. The facilities that are provided and the organisation and administration of the individual specialist's work are costly and the fees charged are consequently high.

CLINICS AND GROUPS

To save costs and enhance quality through the sharing of staff expenses and facilities, some specialists work in groups or from a clinic, and the size of these groups varies from a handful of physicians up to fifty or more. The form of organisation varies also. Many are privately inspired and organised, whilst others are part of a community project such as the Kaiser Permanente Scheme in California, and the Health Insurance Plan in New York. There are some that are part of a Trade Union service for its members such as the Community Health Association in Detroit.

The medical clinic may be a very large group of specialists providing ambulatory care, and a special feature of such clinics is that it is associated closely with a number of local hospitals.

Examples of this are seen in the Mayo Clinic in Rochester, Minnesota, and the Lee Clinic in Palo Alto, California.

The Mayo Clinic is not only a regional centre for specialist ambulatory care but also a medical centre of national and international repute. It has more than 2,000 physicians working in it, of whom 600 are staff members, the others trainees, assistants or associates. It functions primarily as a diagnostic centre for difficult problems. The work of the Mayo Clinic itself is entirely with ambulatory patients but it has the closest relations with the two large local privately owned hospitals to which patients requiring hopitalisation are sent and where the staff of the Mayo Clinic have full access and privileges.

The Lee Clinic at Palo Alto with a medical staff membership of 100 specialists and 6 family physicians provides total and comprehensive care for a population of 110,000 from a single central unit. This demonstrates that it is possible to provide such a service for such a large population.

HOSPITAL OUT-PATIENT SERVICES

For the sizeable proportion of US citizens who cannot meet costs of private specialist services, ambulatory care from specialists is available at out-patient clinics at the larger hospitals, to which the patients have direct access. Much of this work is unpaid and recognised as a voluntary and charitable act on the part of the specialist, and there is a general feeling that this service is for medical indigents only and that as such, it may be of a second-rate quality.

The Specialist in the UK

In the UK, under the NHS, specialist services for ambulatory patients are provided at the out-patient departments of hospitals (OPD). There is in addition a small amount of private practice by which specialists see referred patients in their consulting rooms, outside the NHS, and for which they receive fees from the patient, but such private consultations account for less than 5 per cent of all work in this field.

HISTORICAL BACKGROUND

Originally the hospital was a refuge and shelter for the sick poor, and the medical care available in the seventeenth and eighteenth centuries was considered more effective and safer given at home than in the hospital.

It was only when, because of increased knowledge and specialisation, hospitals became specialised as expert diagnostic and therapeutic units that referral and admission to hospitals became socially more acceptable. At the same time an increase of the population and migration to live in the cities, during the industrial revolution, created a situation where many could not find or afford a private physician.

To provide care for the ambulatory and needy sick, British voluntary hospitals in the late nineteenth and early twentieth centuries created out-patient departments where such patients could be seen free of charge, or on payment of a nominal sum.

Soon the out-patient service became divided into casualty department and the specialist out-patient clinics. The former, staffed by junior doctors or local general practitioners, acted as a hospital unit for accidents and other emergencies, but which also provided general practice care for the sick poor. The specialist clinics dealt with more specific problems and disease groups, and were available to self-referred as well as physician-referred patients.

With the introduction of the NHS in 1948, the out-patient department expanded for two reasons. First, because the general practitioner was excluded from the hospitals to which he previously had access, he began to refer more patients to OPD as the trend for more and more investigations occurred with the growth of medical knowledge. Second, private general practice was reduced greatly and patients became more ready and anxious to see the specialist at a hospital clinic free of charge than in his private consulting rooms for a fee. The old stigma of the OPD being reserved for the poor and needy disappeared.

THE FUNCTIONS AND FEATURES OF THE OUT-PATIENT SERVICE

The out-patient department is an integral and highly developed part of the hospital structure, and provides a consultation service by specialist physicians appointed by the Regional Hospital Boards.

These specialists are chosen as a result of competitive selection and their appointments, in the case of clinicians, include work both in the out-patient and the in-patient hospital departments. There is no differentiation of staff between these two parts of the service (as in the USSR), and as a general rule the physician who first sees the patient in the out-patient department is also responsible for him when he is admitted to the hospital ward.

Patients are only seen by referral from their general practitioners, and there is no direct access by the patient to these specialist ambulatory services.

The specialists are free to organise their work as they wish, within practical limits. They are paid by sessional fees and each consulting session is intended to last 2–3 hours. During this period patients are seen by appointment, and the numbers of new and old patients can be controlled on the specialists' instructions. This may lead to delays and waiting lists for appointments and whilst some clinics have no waiting periods, there are delays for up to 4–6 weeks for certain clinics in orthopaedic, gynaecological and dermatological units in some areas. The disposal of the patients attending the out-patient departments follows a common pattern. (Table 18.)

TABLE 18

Disposal of patients attending out-patient departments on first occasion

	%
Returned to care of GP	20–25
Reattending OPD clinic	45–50
Referred to other OPD clinic	5–10
Placed on waiting list for admission to hospital	20–25

(Source: McLachlan, G. (ed.). *Problems and Progress in Medical Care*, London (1966).)

Of those who reattend the clinic, many do so for reassessment following certain diagnostic investigations, but after this they are returned to the care of their general practitioner.

Hospital out-patient departments do not, as a rule, carry out long-term follow-up of patients, and only 15 per cent of first attenders in the study quoted were still under out-patient care after six months.

Facilities are available at hospital for social welfare from medical social workers, who are quite separate and distinct from the community social workers employed by the local public health authorities (see Chapter 8).

The out-patient department serves as the local diagnostic centre for general practitioners, and the majority have direct and open access for their patients to the pathology and radiology departments. General practitioners may refer their patients to these diagnostic departments for investigations to be carried out, and the results to be sent back directly to the general practitioners.

Minor surgical procedures are carried out in some out-patient clinics, such as ligation of varicose veins and repair of herniae, and the out-patient Department of Physical Medicine may act as the local rehabilitation centre.

UTILISATION

Each year 15–16 per cent of the population of the UK attend hospital out-patient departments as 'new patients', i.e. they are fresh referrals by the general practitioners. (Report of Ministry of Health for 1966.) Another 5–10 per cent are attending follow-up clinics, thus one in five of all Britons attend hospital clinics each year.

The ranking of clinic usage, by numbers seen, is shown in Table 19.

TABLE 19

New patients referred as percentage of population at risk, England and Wales

Out-patient clinic	New patients percentage of population
1. Orthopaedic and trauma	2·2
2. General surgical	2·0
3. Ear, nose and throat	1·4
4. Ophthalmic	1·3
5. General medical	1·3
6. Chest diseases	0·9
7. Dermatology	0·8

(Source: Report of Ministry of Health for 1966.)

Table 20 shows the numbers of patients who are seen in each clinic, which is usually staffed by a specialist with one or two medical assistants. It illustrates the differing patterns of work in the various specialities and these differences are demonstrated further in Table 21 where the average time spent per patient is shown.

Direct Comparisons of Specialist Care for the Ambulatory Patient

Between the three countries the understanding of the term 'specialist' differs. Thus in the UK the specialist who is

TABLE 20

Mean numbers per clinic of new and old patients attending
out-patient clinics in England and Wales

Speciality	New patients (new attenders)	Old patients (reattenders)	Total
General medical	4·3	17·5	21·8
Paediatric	4·0	12·9	16·9
General surgical	7·7	18·6	26·3
ENT	10·2	21·4	31·6
Orthopaedic	9·3	27·7	37·0
Gynaecological	8·5	14·5	23·0
Obstetrics			
Antenatal	6·5	32·4	38·9
Postnatal	13·1	2·0	15·1
Psychiatric	1·1	6·2	7·3

Patients were seen by a specialist and 1 or 2 assistants.
(Sources: Annual Reports of Ministry of Health.)

TABLE 21

Times for consultations for new and old (reattenders)
patients in the UK out-patient departments

Speciality	Average time per consultation	
	New patients (min.)	Old patients (min.)
General medical	25	9
Paediatric	18	8
General surgical	10	8
ENT	7	6
Orthopaedic	10	7
Fracture clinic	5	4
Gynaecological	12	8
Obstetrics	6	5
Psychiatric	27	13

(Source: *Waiting in Out Patient Departments*, Nuffield
Provincial Hospitals Trust, London (1963).)

responsible for out-patient care in hospitals is appointed
competitively after a lengthy training and examinations, and
he only sees patients referred to him by general practitioners,
whilst in the USA there is no clear distinction between the
specialist and the 'specialoid' and it is left to the patient to
decide whom to consult. In the USSR the polyclinic specialist

occupies an intermediate position between the doctor-of-first-contact and the consultant specialist, as recognised in the UK. The polyclinic specialist does not work in hospital and he is responsible for only a small population, that covered by the polyclinic (less than 50,000).

In all three countries although most of the care is carried out in the physicians' consulting rooms or clinic, some home visits are carried out.

In the USSR all polyclinic specialists are expected to visit any patients who are housebound and under their care, and the numbers of such home visits are set out by the norms and standards of the Ministry of Health. In the UK there is a special scheme, the 'domiciliary consultation scheme', whereby a general practitioner may call in a specialist to a patient at home when that patient is too sick to attend the hospital out-patient department, but in the USA although it is possible for a specialist to carry out home visiting, it is nevertheless very unusual.

It is only in the UK that full and free access of patients to specialists is restricted, and they can be seen by specialists in the out-patient departments only through referral by their general practitioners. In both the USSR and the USA patients can choose when and which specialist they wish to see.

In the United Kingdom the out-patient service that provides specialist ambulatory care is a part of the hospital service and the specialists who see out-patients also care for them when they are admitted to hospital, but there is separation of urban polyclinics from hospitals in the USSR and polyclinic specialists do not provide continuing care for patients who are admitted to hospital.

By contrast almost all specialists in the USA have access to hospital beds and continue to care for their patients in hospital.

With regard to diagnostic facilities the specialist in private practice in the USA has to provide his own or else refer his patients to private diagnostic clinics, but in the UK and the USSR all specialist diagnostic facilities are available freely and readily either in the hospital (UK) or in the polyclinic (USSR).

Any comparison of the numbers of specialists working in the ambulatory care field is difficult, and these difficulties arise from the differing roles and functions of the specialists.

For example the specialists in Soviet polyclinics are excluded from hospitals, but in the UK they are based in the hospitals, whilst in the USA there is a whole range of possibilities.

Table 22 shows the ratios of various specialists to the populations that they care for in the hospital out-patient and in-patient services in England and Wales.

TABLE 22

Ratios of hospital specialists to population in England and Wales

Speciality	Ratio of specialist to population
General medicine	1 : 59,000
General surgery	1 : 55,000
Dermatology	1 : 250,000
Geriatrics	1 : 250,000
Ophthalmology	1 : 140,000
Neurology	1 : 500,000
Psychiatry	1 : 50,000
ENT	1 : 170,000
Orthopaedics	1 : 110,000
Paediatrics	1 : 200,000
Gynaecology	1 : 67,000
Thoracic surgeons	1 : 500,000
Chest physicians	1 : 140,000
ALL SPECIALITIES	1 : 5,300

Note: UK specialists undertake in-patient duties in addition to care of ambulatory patients at out-patient departments.
(Source: Report of Ministry of Health for 1966.)

In the USSR the ratio of polyclinic specialists to population served is quite different as shown in Table 23.

Comparison of Tables 22 and 23 suggests that there are ten times as many specialists in the USSR as in the UK but the understanding of what is meant by a 'specialist' is different. The clinical experience of the specialist in the UK for example, is derived from a population 10 times that of the Soviet specialist.

TABLE 23

Ratios of specialists to population in
USSR polyclinics

Speciality	Ratio of specialist to population
General medicine	1 : 2,500
General surgery	1 : 8,000
Dermatology (and VD)	1 : 17,000
Ophthalmology	1 : 20,000
Neurology (and psychiatry)	1 : 20,000
ENT	1 : 17,000
Paediatrics	1 : 4,000
Gynaecology	1 : 8,000
Tuberculosis	1 : 8,000
ALL SPECIALITIES	1 : 550

Note: Polyclinic specialists do not have
hospital duties.
(Source: Popov, G.A. 1967.)

A Personal Evaluation

Specialist services for ambulatory patients represent an essential level in the flow of medical care. Being placed between first-contact care and the hospital, they serve as a link between these two parts of medical care and have certain special roles and features.

To function effectively physicians working in this field must be specialists. That is to say that they must have received a recognised training, with assessment and tests of their ability, in a special branch of medical care. Once qualified as a specialist, the physician must have the opportunity to increase his experience by working with pre-selected clinical material in his own branch of medical or surgical care. Direct access to specialists by the public is therefore undesirable because the ordinary man-in-the-street cannot be expected to select the correct specialist for his symptoms; a system of referral between physicians is necessary.

The specialist will work with, and become experienced in, the rarer and the more complex forms of disease, but to become so experienced and reach a high quality he must have responsibility for a population large enough to supply

I

such cases. A decision has to be made on the size of population that will provide the various specialists with sufficient numbers of cases, and at the same time provide a satisfactory public service.

How many gastric operations does the surgeon require to perform each year to maintain his skills? How many cases of diabetic coma does a physician require to provide a good service? Such questions need careful thought and the problems need careful analysis.

The specialist can become and remain an expert only if he has access to modern diagnostic and therapeutic equipment. Where should such equipment be available to ensure both economy and availability?

Expensive equipment has to be centralised so that it may be used frequently and regularly by many and it is uneconomic, for example, to have a modern radiology unit or pathology laboratory serving less than 100,000 persons.

In these circumstances specialist services must be concentrated in centres that serve populations large enough to warrant the basing of specialists in such units, and capable of providing them with enough material.

The alternatives are to site the ambulatory specialist services either at a local district hospital or at a community medical clinic. In either case the population cared for should be well over 50,000 and probably more than 100,000, if the specialists are to be employed effectively. Alternatively the specialist may visit smaller units at regular but infrequent intervals.

Wherever the specialist services are sited there must be good relations and communications with first-contact services and hospitals. The first-contact service has the function of protecting the specialist from non-specialist problems and the hospital has to provide the extra facilities required to manage the conditions facing him. It seems undeniably necessary, therefore, for the ambulatory specialist to work in the hospital.

Chapter 6
Hospitals

Hospitals are the most expensive and the most specialised part of the modern medical care system. They cannot function effectively in isolation and without collaboration from the first-contact and ambulatory specialist services, they fulfil several specific roles in the community. The hospital provides in-patient care, out-patient service and acts as a diagnostic centre.

In extending the concept that the hospital is the chief local diagnostic and therapeutic centre, it follows that the hospital should act also as the local centre for the medical profession, providing graduate and post-graduate educational facilities not only for physicians, but for all para-medical workers.

The Hospitals of the USSR

The close inter-relationship of central and local planning in Soviet Russia has led to a common national policy of hospital building and development, that is nevertheless adaptable to local factors andrequirements.

Uchastok Hospital (*Local General Hospital*)

This is the smallest hospital unit, and usually serves sparsely populated rural areas the local hospital providing care for 2,000 to 15,000 persons. They are completely integrated with the polyclinic, sharing the same premises and having a common medical and nursing staff. The physicians work as a team combining hospital, specialist and first-contact care.

This team comprises paediatrician; therapist (general physician for adults); surgeon, who also undertakes gynae-

Hospitals

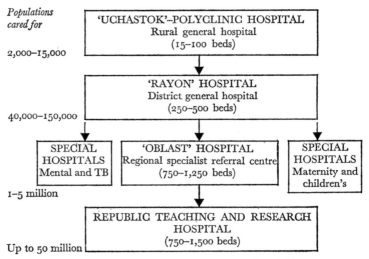

Fig. 12. Structure of hospital system in the USSR.

cology and obstetrics; and a dental surgeon. In the larger units there also will be a radiologist and pathologist.

The local hospital–polyclinic works with a number of 'feldsher–midwife' posts situated in villages or collective farms and they are under the supervision of the physicians in the parent hopital–polyclinic. Such local hospitals range in size from 15 to 100 beds, but the present trend is to close those with less than 50 beds.

The work carried out in these small hospitals is principally for traumatic and surgical emergencies; acute medical conditions, such as chest infections, rheumatic fever and peptic ulcers; some chronic disorders such as degenerative arthritis and strokes; and normal obstetrics.

Such small units have few resources for the care of more major conditions and a close relationship exists with the District and the Regional hospitals. Specialists from these larger hospitals are often called in by the physicians working in the local unit to assist them in making a diagnosis and in carrying out surgical operations.

A medical air-transport service covers the whole of the USSR and patients can easily be moved to larger and more expert units or specialists can be brought by air to the patient within a few hours.

DISTRICT HOSPITAL

These are typical district general hospitals, staffed and equipped for dealing with most cases except those requiring highly specialised care. Serving populations of from 40,000 to 150,000 there is often more than one such hospital in each large District, and the largest one is referred to as the Central Hospital which acts as the district's medical administrative centre. They are associated with a number of polyclinics, one of which may be sited in the hospital grounds.

The medical staff of the District hospital is separate from that of the polyclinics and is not involved in work outside the hospital. There are no general clinics at the hospital for ambulatory patients, it is for in-patients only.

Admission into hospital is through the polyclinics, there being no self-referral by patients.

The existing District hospitals tend to be between 250 and 500 beds, but the future trends are for larger hospitals of 1,000–1,200 beds.

The basic divisions of care are medical, surgical, obstetric-gynaecological (but this division may be in a separate maternity hospital), paediatric (this also may be in a separate hospital) and infectious diseases. In the larger hospitals there may be additional departments for eye disorders, ear, nose and throat diseases and for orthopaedic surgery. Administratively, there is a Chief Physician who is usually responsible also for all the medical services in the District, including polyclinic and public health services.

The District hospitals work closely with the Regional hospital (*vide infra*), which is the centre for the super-specialities, and complex cases are referred there, or specialists from it may be brought in.

THE REGIONAL HOSPITAL

This functions as the regional specialist centre for a population of 1–5 million. Acting as a referral centre from the Districts it does not, as a rule, admit patients directly from the community or the polyclinics. It has no system of out-patient clinics, although some of its departments do follow up their patients after discharge from hospitals.

Hospital

Regional hospitals are intended to be large and contain 750–1,250 beds. Specialities such as neurosurgery, chest and heart surgery and most radiotherapy are centred there, but they also have general medical and surgical units which deal with the more complex conditions, such as skeletal tuberculosis, rheumatic heart disease and haematology. Each clinical department is headed by a chief physician who in addition to his work and responsibilities at the Regional hospital is responsible also for the planning, organisation and quality of his speciality's services in the whole region.

Thus, the chief surgeon at the Regional hospital organises and supervises surgical services throughout all the District hospitals and polyclinics in the region. He is assisted in this by a committee who carry out regular visits to District hospitals and polyclinics and by constant critical analysis of the records of work carried out at the more peripheral units. The Regional hospital is the centre for postgraduate studies and research and specialists working in the periphery come for courses and meetings and most research projects are undertaken at the Regional level.

THE REPUBLIC HOSPITAL

At the apex of the hospital hierarchical pyramid is the Republic Hospital.

This institution acts as Regional hospital in that it serves as regional specialist centre, but it is also a *medical institute*, the teaching medical school for undergraduate education.

The republic hospital complex may incorporate more than one hospital and the teaching of undergraduates may be dispersed in a number of units. In addition to acting as a medical school the Republic hospital may incorporate one or more 'scientific research institutes' which are special recognised research units undertaking work in a specific topic or subject. These scientific research institutes are associated with the Central USSR Academy of Medical Sciences in Moscow.

SPECIAL HOSPITALS

Mental hospitals are not part of the general hospital structure. They function separately on a District or Regional basis with their own buildings for in-patients and their own dispensaries, or out-patient, units, providing thus a full area service for mental illness. Patients have direct access to the psychiatric dispensary in the community and this serves as a special polyclinic caring for ambulatory cases. It also functions as a day-hospital and as the follow-up clinic for patients after discharge from hospital.

Care for the tuberculous is on similar lines. The District tuberculosis dispensary usually incorporates a hospital unit with beds, a polyclinic, a sanatorium for convalescent patients and sheltered workshops for after-care and rehabilitation.

Maternity hospitals may be part of the District hospital, but in large cities they are separate and associated closely with the Women's Consultation Clinics.

The same applies to Children's hospitals which may be separate or alternatively a unit or division in a District hospital.

HOSPITAL ADMINISTRATION (see also Chapter 3)

All top hospital administrators in the USSR are physicians. Not only are they physicians but they are practising clinicians who combine medical administration with their clinical work.

This principle of part-time administration extends right through the Soviet medical system from the Minister of Health, who always has been a practising physician, to the medical administrators of District and Local hospitals.

Medical administration is a competitive extra which receives additional remuneration, and suitable selected candidates undergo a 3–6 months period of special training in medical administration before taking up their appointments.

THE FUNCTION OF THE SOVIET HOSPITAL

Soviet hospitals are primarily, and almost solely, in-patient units caring for those patients who require hospitalisation. Ambulatory patients who require specialist care, advice and follow-up are seen in the polyclinics which are distinct from the urban hospitals. It is the polyclinics that serve as the main diagnostic centres within the community, with the

Hospitals

District hospital's laboratories and radiology units supplementing these diagnostic resources.

The hospital's contacts with the community are through the polyclinics. Apart from special hospitals, as for tuberculosis, psychiatry and obstetrics, which have their own associate polyclinics, there is no recognisable community role for the general hospital. Hospitals act as local professional medical centres engaged in continuing education. The District hospitals have regular exchanges of medical staff with the polyclinics for educational purposes, and for three months every year the less senior staff of the polyclinics and the District hospital exchange appointments.

The Regional hospital has a more specific educational role and offers special facilities for higher professional training as well as refresher courses.

RELATIONS WITH OTHER BRANCHES

There are good and easy relations and contacts between hospitals at the various levels. Specialists proceed from Regional hospital to District and Local hospitals for advice and assistance and there are no difficulties in transferring a patient from one hospital to another.

Relations between hospitals and polyclinics are less easy in practice than in theory for with separate staffs and administration any relations are on a formal basis and communications are more through correspondence than by personal contact.

Links with the public health services also tend to be at the more formal levels. The two systems are distinct, but the local public health department does have certain duties to ensure compliance by the hospital with public health measures and the two do come together in matters of public health policy involving early diagnosis.

PLANNING AND BUILDING

Hospital planning is based on the national system of indicators, norms and standards, which are decided by the Ministry of Health of the USSR as the result of continuing studies and surveys. Considerable flexibility is applied to meet local conditions. Planning of hospital services corresponds with national five-year plans of general production and economic growth, and all such exercises begin locally at the District hospital level being the responsibility of the chief physician assisted by a committee. Local hospital plans are then submitted up through the various higher levels for co-ordination and costing and final approval rests with the Ministry of Health of the USSR.

The building of hospitals has been developed to fit national plans with the use of standard modules and extensive application of prefabrication. It is estimated that more than 90 per cent of hospitals in the USSR are now of the 'standard' type. With such standardisation and prefabrication building times have been speeded up and it is claimed that it is possible now to complete the planning and building of a 1,000-bed general hospital in eighteen months.

The quality of the new hospitals can be described only as fair. The general design of hospitals is old-fashioned. Concentration on small ward units of 1–4 beds and day-rooms nevertheless has created a curious impression of lack of space. Operating theatres often open directly on to corridors, making sterility difficult and ancillary rooms are limited. As with most modern Soviet buildings the standard of finish is poor and paintwork and door and window fittings deteriorate quickly. In recent times, however, there has been a need to place quantity and speed of building, before sophistication of design.

RESOURCES AND UTILISATION

In the USSR in 1966 there were 9.6 hospital beds per 1,000 population, varying from 8.1 in Soviet Armenia to 11.6 per 1,000 in Soviet Latvia. This figure of 9.6 per 1,000 includes only 0.93 per 1,000 hospital beds for mental illnesses, a very much lower rate than in the USA and the UK, where such resources are four times greater. This availability of 9.6 beds per 1,000 is considered too low and the target 'norm' for the future is 11.2 beds per 1,000 for general conditions plus 2.0 per 1,000 for mental illnesses, and thus in effect it is proposed to double the proportion of hospital beds for mental illnesses.

Hospitals

In addition there are many beds in convalescent homes ('sanatoria') which are used either for continuing care of some chronic illnesses or for purely rehabilitative, convalescent or holiday purposes. The proposed norms for hospitals and sanatoria are shown in Table 24.

TABLE 24
Proposed 'norms' for hospital beds in the USSR

Speciality	Hospital beds	Sanatoria convalescent homes
	Per 1,000	Per 1,000
General medicine	2·2	0·97
General surgery	1·9	0·5
Obstetrics	1·1	0·25
Gynaecology	0·9	0·25
Neurology	0·3	0·6
Psychiatry	2·0	—
Paediatrics	1·2	0·2
Infectious diseases	1·4	—
Tuberculosis	1·2	0·2
Ophthalmology	0·35	—
ENT	0·25	—
Skin and VD	0·4	0·05
TOTAL	13·2	3·02

(Source: Popov, G.A., and others, personal communications, 1967.)

HOSPITAL UTILISATION

In 1965 more than 40 million (out of 230 million) Soviet citizens were hospitalised. This represented rates of 20 per cent of the urban and 18 per cent of the rural populations. The average length of stay in hospital was 15–16 days and the annual level of bed occupancy was 85 per cent.

PERSONNEL

There are no figures readily available of the numbers of medical and paramedical staff that are actually working in Soviet hospitals.

According to Popov (1967) (*Efficiency of Medical Care*, WHO, Regional Office for Europe), the 'norms' for 100 hospital beds are 9 *physicians*, including: general medicine 0.97, paediatrics 0.92 gynaecology and obstetrics 1.2 and general surgery 0.8.

This means that approximately one-third of all physicians in the USSR are working in hospitals; providing care for in-patients only. The stated 'norm' for *paramedical staff* is 38.04 per 100 hospital beds, including 30.75 nurses, 4.55 midwives and 1.53 laboratory technicians. (See also Chapter 11.)

QUALITY INDICES

Certain criteria are used to endeavour to estimate the quality of work in hospitals.

The quality indices used include the following:

1. The average length of patient stay in each department, the annual work load, bed occupancy, and turnover.
2. The 'timeliness' of emergency surgical aid, i.e. how soon admitted from onset of symptoms.
3. The volume and range of surgical work.
4. Rates of complications in surgical and obstetric departments.
5. Death rates in hospitals with special reference to post-operative, maternal and infant mortality.
6. Accuracy of correlation between clinical and morbid-anatomical diagnoses.

The final quality assessment of a hospital is made by a summation of these indices, and due allowances are made for local factors such as general morbidity and mortality of the population and the age structure. These qualitative indices are used to compare individual hospitals and units and also for the planning and developing future services. Recently (1965/66) a number of research studies have been carried out by the Semashko Institute of Moscow into the city's hospital care. Among its findings were that up to 12 per cent of all hospital patients in Moscow were there unnecessarily and could be transferred easily to convalescent homes – this proportion of 'needless' hospital patients was as high as 30 per cent in general medical and general surgical departments.

Emergency Care Services

In the USSR there is an impressive system of emergency care service, which is organised on a nation-wide scale with close links and integration between ambulance services, polyclinics and hospitals.

It is a free service. It is accessible widely, using all forms of transport including land, sea and air; prevention is an integral part of its work; and the public is actively involved through health education and first-aid training.

The prime objective of the emergency services is to provide 'maximal available coverage', implying an extension of the hospital-type intensive care to the patient at the site of the accident.

The work includes:

1. Transport of emergency and planned hospital admissions.
2. Admission of pregnant women.
3. First-aid for, and the management of, accidents and sudden emergencies.
4. Special ambulance units for cardiac emergencies, shock, severe trauma, neurological emergencies and mentally disturbed patients.
5. Participation in research and prevention of accidents.
6. Education and training of the public in first-aid.
7. Community Medical Information Centre.

In large cities (where more than 25,000 calls are dealt with each year) the ambulance service is organised as an independent unit with its own centralised administration. In the smaller towns the ambulances are attached to local polyclinics and hospitals and in rural areas each polyclinic–hospital has its own ambulances.

There is one ambulance to 10.000 persons in urban areas and one to 15,000 in rural areas.

A special feature of the Soviet emergency care services is the considerable number of medical and paramedical staff. Thus in Kiev, a city of $1\frac{1}{4}$ millions, the central ambulance station has its own full-time staff of 300 physicians and 400 'feldshers' and nurses.

AMBULANCE TEAMS

The type of ambulance and team sent to an incident

depends on the skill of the central emergency organisation. The public has direct communicative contact with the ambulance station and trained telephone operators accept incoming calls and translate them into the necessary action required. This unit also acts as an information centre for missing persons and for general advice on lay medical problems and procedures. For routine transport of the sick the ambulance is a modified large limousine with space for a stretcher and the team sent to normal cases consists of a driver and two feldshers.

For accidents and medical emergencies, however, the team comprises a physician, a 'feldsher' and a driver and emergency ambulances designed to provide 'maximal coverage' are available for specific situations. Specially trained 'cardiac' teams are ready to deal with heart cases, particularly those associated with myocardial infarction. Such an ambulance will be staffed by one cardiologist and four technicians, and the ambulance will be equipped with an electrocardiograph, defibrillator, equipment for pathological tests and surgical procedures, an anaesthetic machine and drugs. In Kiev there are two such ambulances and they have resuscitated twenty cases of cardiac arrest in the past two years.

Special ambulance units are also available for major trauma, shock, obstetric and psychiatric emergencies.

FLYING DOCTORS

There are many helicopter ambulance units in rural areas for transport of the sick and to take specialists to outlying hospitals.

FUTURE TRENDS

Certain general trends are notable in the Soviet hospital system.

Following a period of tremendous growth with more emphasis on quantity than on quality, there is now appreciation that better utilisation must be made of existing facilities rather than a policy of blind and uncritical expansion. The study referred to in Moscow by the Semashko Institute, for example, which showed a high rate of 'needless' hospitalisation is being used as evidence for better rationalisation of hospital usage. At the same time the planners are predicting the need for more hospital beds as the population becomes older and as more emphasis is placed on the extension of 'preventive hospitalisation'. It is anticipated that the eventual requirements will be to meet annual admission rates of 24 per cent of the total population, and to meet such rates the norms of hospital beds are being increased to 13.2 per 1,000.

The reasons for such a high rate of hospitalisation is the Soviet custom of admitting patients with common clinical disorders, that in the UK would certainly be managed at home, and the belief that in many situations early admission serves a preventive purpose by avoiding progressive deterioration in conditions such as peptic ulcers, hypertension and chronic rheumatism. There is no supportive evidence forthcoming or available for such a hypothesis. A typical example of this Soviet approach is that during recent influenza epidemics vulnerable patients with chronic chest ailments and heart conditions were admitted prophylactically to hospital.

The future policy, however, is to have larger general hospitals of 1,000–1,200 beds with 'diversification', and this means that there will be more special units within general hospitals. In large cities this diversification policy will lead to the establishment of more special hospitals, separate and apart from general hospitals in order to concentrate care for specific problems.

A high priority in the USSR is to improve the hospital facilities in those rural areas which are recognised as being less well served than those in urban areas, and as part of this exercise many small rural hospitals with less than fifty beds are being replaced by larger units.

The Hospitals of the USA

Historically, the earliest 'hospitals' in the USA were almshouses for the sick–poor and isolation hospitals at seaports designed for quarantine protection against contagious diseases.

The first general hospital was built at Philadelphia in 1751, and hospital building, since it relied on voluntary funds, was slow until the immigration explosion of the early twentieth century. From 1900 to 1940 there was an era of tremendous building of new hospitals, but relying on local initiatives and wealth this was haphazard and unplanned, being unrelated to the real social and medical needs. It was in 1946 as a result of the findings of a Commission on Hospital Care sponsored by the American Hospital Association and the Federal Public Health Service that the Hill-Burton Act (the Hospital Survey and Construction Act) was passed. The basic philosophy of this legislation was that health was a national resource and that Federal leadership and finance were necessary to establish an adequate network of hospital and related facilities, and the States were encouraged to undertake planning of hospital building, based on careful inventories of existing facilities.

In spite of the Hill-Burton Act and the more recent advent of Medicare and Medicaid, and other legislation, the US hospital services are still organised in a laissez-faire and independent fashion. A lack of co-ordinated planning in the past, in spite of the terms of the Hill-Burton Act, has resulted in the irregular distribution of hospitals and even in certain areas a degree of competition for patients between them. Hospitals have tended also to become 'status symbols' with the result that there are many small hospitals with superfluous resources.

TYPES OF HOSPITALS IN THE USA

There is no simple recognisable pattern of American hospitals. They cannot be graded readily according to populations served or size or roles, because there is so much overlap.

TABLE 25

Types of US hospitals and the proportions of their numbers and beds

Type of hospital	Percentage of total hospitals	Percentage of total hospital beds	Average number of beds per hospital
Federal	6	10	400
State	8	42	1,280
Local government	21	13	140
Church	17	13	175
Non-profit voluntary	34	19	130
Proprietary	14	3	55
	100(= 7,127)	100(= 1·7 million)	—

(Source: US Bureau of the Census, *U.S.A. 1967*.)

A useful classification however is according to their type, and Table 25 shows the proportions of these.

Federal Hospitals (6 per cent of hospitals and 10 per cent of beds) include military hospitals, those of the Veterans Administration and those of the Public Health Service. They tend to be large with an average of 400 beds per hospital and the staff are all full-time federal employees. Many are of a very high professional standard.

State Hospitals (8 per cent of hospitals and 42 per cent of beds) are owned and administered by the various states. They care for chronic sick, including mental illnesses and tuberculosis, and they are very large with an average size of more than 1,000 beds, staffed by full-time state employees. The quality of care in these State hospitals is variable and they tend to be understaffed in both nurses and physicians.

Local Government Hospitals (21 per cent of hospitals and 13 per cent of beds) are owned and administered by local municipalities and counties these are the district general hospital for the medical indigents, those who cannot afford the fees of the private hospitals. They provide general care for acute and chronic illnesses and there are also special local government hospitals for specific conditions. Staffed by a mixture of full-time and part-time personnel they range in size from 1,000 to 20 beds, with an average of 140 beds per hospital. Most are modern with good facilities and standards of care.

Voluntary Church Hospitals (17 per cent of hospitals and 13 per cent of beds) are a separate category because of their large number – 17 per cent of all hospitals. Apart from the fact that they are owned by religious denominations they are in effect 'voluntary non-profit' hospitals, and they rely on voluntary contributions and fees for their funds but they are not profit-making. The medical staffs comprise local physicians who are either specially appointed in some areas or who are all allowed access in other places. The medical staff may include therefore an almost unlimited number of physicians (one Californian hospital of 300 beds has over 800 physicians on its staff), or be restricted to a set number. All patients must pay fees both to the hospital and to the physicians.

Voluntary Non-profit Community Hospitals (34 per cent

of hospitals and 19 per cent of beds) account for one-third of all hospitals, and together with the Church-owned hospitals for one-half. They range from large and world-renowned *teaching hospitals* associated with universities to *local community hospitals* of no more than 10–20 beds. Most of them are general hospitals with an average of 130 beds, but lacking or only possessing few speciality beds, although they offer full privileges for local physicians. The teaching hospitals are affiliated to local medical schools and the staff are all specially appointed specialists with a staff of junior physicians.

Proprietary Hospitals (14 per cent of hospitals and 3 per cent of beds) are small (average 55 beds), privately-owned, established, administered and organised to make profits for their owners or shareholders. They offer facilities to all physicians, but because of their small size these facilities tend to be limited.

Not fitting into these categories are hospitals owned and administered by Trade Unions and other organisations, which combine features of the government and non-government hospitals.

SPECIAL FEATURES OF HOSPITALS IN THE USA

In the voluntary and proprietary hospitals (but not in university and public ones) open access to beds and other facilities for all local physicians who satisfy certain criteria (these do not exclude many physicians) is a characteristic of the American hospital pattern. This leads to a large visiting 'staff' – each member of which may have only one or two patients in the hospital at one time, and the nursing staff has many 'bosses' and many habits of therapy to cope with. Once given hospital access and privileges, the physicians can undertake a wide area of care, and they may handle rare conditions very infrequently.

In some areas, particularly the more prosperous, competition for patients exists between local hospitals, since lack of regional and national planning has led to an excess of hospital facilities in some localities. In such circumstances hospital administrators are encouraged to use public relations officers and other means of self advertisement such as statements in local newspapers when a prominent person

K

enters a particular hospital. This competition also leads to certain hospital 'status symbols', where features such as the possession of a computer; the possession of a 'cobalt bomb' unit; the ability to perform open heart surgery albeit infrequently; and the listing of a neurosurgeon on the staff are all current symbols of status in the eyes of certain groups of the public. Even small hospitals of 150–200 beds may consider such features as necessities.

Because open access exists for all local physicians, quality controls have become an important part of American hospital life, and various committees are set up to undertake this form of assessment. 'Accreditation committees' from outside the hospital assess the work of the hospital as a whole, whilst 'tissue committees', from within the hospital, examine material removed at surgical operations and assess whether operations may have been unnecessary. In the USA the rate of litigation and claims for malpraxis is much greater than in the UK at present (no figures are available from the USSR) and this factor in itself has led to the institution of many quality controls and professional safeguards.

'Waiting lists' for admission to hospital do not exist in the USA as they do in the UK. This, presumably, is because the numbers of hospital beds are at present keeping pace with the demand (to be distinguished from 'needs' and 'wants') of those covered by pre-paid insurance or able to afford private fees. In some areas, as in California, the occupancy rates of the proprietary and voluntary hospitals runs at 75 per cent or less, signifying a surfeit of beds and explaining the competition for patients. The remarkably short stays of many patients in American hospitals may be explained by the fact that many are admitted for diagnostic and minor procedures in order to meet insurance-cover requirements.

The supply of trained nurses in the United States has not kept pace with the growth of hospitals and the development of medical science and it is particularly short in the middle nursing grades. The numbers of top-level nursing administrators are adequate as are those of nursing graduates who carry out many technical tasks; but there are shortages amongst practical nurses to carry out personal nursing and less technical duties.

The costs of hospital care are rising steeply. Since the introduction of Medicare legislation these costs have risen even more steeply, possibly because the 'government' is now to meet many of the bills. Some three out of four of the population are covered for hospital costs through pre-paid insurance schemes, excluding those under Medicare provisions and such insurance cover profoundly influences the customs and habits of hospital care. Thus, because these schemes do not meet the costs of investigations for patients not in hospital, many are admitted for short periods merely so that these costs can be recovered. In a recent publication (*Custom and Practice in Medical Care* (Simpson, J., Mair, A., Thomas, R.G., Willard, H.N., and Bakst, H.J., London, 1968)), a close comparison is made of a British and an American hospital, and from this study it becomes clear how short 'diagnostic' admissions account for many of the hospital admissions in the USA. Since firstly physicians are paid by fees-for-services and those for the hospital care of patients are appreciably higher than for care outside hospital – and secondly since most persons are insured only for hospital care, then inevitably there is encouragement for physicians to admit patients readily and so claim the higher fees paid by the insurance companies.

In general most US hospitals are well equipped with good premises and comfortable facilities for the patient. This applies particularly to the voluntary non-profit and proprietary hospitals and whilst standards in State and local government hospitals are less elaborate they are still high by any standards.

URBAN AND RURAL DIFFERENCES

There are major differences in quality and resources between urban and rural hospitals, and there is no close link between the rural and the city hospitals. No standard system is evident whereby specialists or experts can come quickly to outlying hospitals in emergencies, and the physicians in small rural hospitals, who are independent and self-reliant, tend to undertake more complex procedures than in similar hospitals in the USSR or the UK. There are medical staff shortages in rural areas and it has become difficult to attract physicians and nurses from the cities to the country.

Hospitals

On account of the emphasis on free enterprise and independence of action, overall planning of hospital services in the USA has been difficult and the results unremarkable. Attempts have been made since the Hill-Burton Act of 1946 to plan regionally but it is only in the past few years that any real progress has been made, by the setting up of Regional Planning Groups with federal support and funds. With three-quarters of the American population covered by pre-paid insurance for hospital care the power of insurance groups such as 'Blue Cross' has increased and they are now able to influence hospital planning, organisation, administration and quality controls. Another important influence in planning is the American Hospitals Association to which most non-government hospitals belong. This association has been concerned with improving the quality of care through various controls and standards and it is now becoming increasingly involved with a more rational programme of hospital planning.

In 1964 there were 8.9 beds per 1,000 of the US population but this proportion has fallen since 1950 because of reductions in the numbers of beds for mental illnesses and tuberculosis. (US Bureau of the Census, *U.S.A. 1967*.) (Table 26.)

TABLE 26

Hospital beds per 1,000 in the USA

	1950	1955	1960	1964
General hospital beds per 1,000	4·5	4·9	4·4	4·7
Psychiatric beds per 1,000	4·6	4·5	4·5	4·0
Tuberculosis beds per 1,000	0·5	0·4	0·3	0·2
Total hospital beds per 1,000	9·6	9·8	9·2	8·9

(Source: US Bureau of the Census, *U.S.A. 1967*.)

In 1964 14.8 per cent of all US citizens were admitted to hospital on one or more occasions and Table 27 shows that the trends since 1950 have been for more persons to be hospitalised each year but for shorter periods.

It is not possible to state how many physicians work in American hospitals because of the varying degrees of access by physicians to their local hospitals. Of all *nurses* 69 per cent work in hospitals in a ratio of 59 nurses per 100 hospital

TABLE 27

US hospitals – utilisation data

	1950	1955	1960	1964
General hospitals				
Annual admissions per 1,000 at risk	110	125	136	145
Average length of stay (days)	10·6	9·9	9·3	9·2
Mental hospitals				
Annual admissions per 1,000	2·0	2·2	2·3	2·7
Average length of stay (days)	83	75	60	50
Tuberculosis hospitals				
Annual admissions per 1,000	0·7	0·7	0·4	0·3
Average length of stay (days)	233	219	200	164
TOTAL ANNUAL ADMISSIONS PER 1,000	113	128	139	148

(Source: US Bureau of the Census, *U.S.A. 1967*.)

beds (*Health Manpower*, 1967, US PHS Publication No. 1667) and of these, 21 are Registered Nurses, 9 are Practical Nurses and 29 are nursing aides.

TRENDS

The chief trend in US hospital care is the increasing rate of hospitalisation; this is rising by 10 per 1,000 every five years.

Yet the beds available have fallen in proportion, for they are being used more effectively and in different ways. This cannot go on continually and steps are being taken to build new hospitals and rebuild old ones – a programme which has been intensified with the increasing demands created by Medicare.

The Hospitals of the UK

The hospital system in the United Kingdom is one of the three parts of the National Health Service (NHS), the other two being general practice and public health services. This tripartite system had existed for generations and the introduction of the NHS merely ensured its continuation.

Originally there were two distinct hospital systems – the voluntary and the municipal – separately organised and financed, and each with its own traditions and fund of experience, and in some ways competing with each other. There were also very definite social associations and images. The municipal hospitals were for the poor and it was considered 'bad taste' for the middle and upper classes to enter them, whilst the voluntary hospitals, who catered for all classes, had private wards for those who wished them.

These voluntary hospitals were independent organisations administered by their own governing bodies, and they varied greatly in size and quality, from the large city general hospitals with modern facilities, to small 'cottage' hospitals of less than fifty beds with very limited resources. They were highly selective in their work and tended to accept only those cases requiring active and short-term treatment, leaving to the municipal hospitals the care of the chronic sick, the elderly, the mentally sick and those suffering from tuberculosis and other infectious diseases. An important difference between the two was that whilst voluntary hospitals, being independent, could refuse to admit a case, municipal hospitals had, by law, to admit all referred to them.

A special group of voluntary hospitals were the Teaching Hospitals, many of which traced their history to the Middle Ages. They were considered the 'best' hospitals with enormous funds, plentiful medical and nursing staff and the loudest voices in the profession. Their medical schools educated students and were affiliated to a university.

Before World War II hospitalisation was not popular, and people were afraid to enter hospital because they considered it was the place where most of those who entered died. The era of scientific advance had not yet arrived. During World War II hospitals were co-ordinated and placed under regional control as part of the Emergency Medical Service, and the differences and discriminations between hospitals vanished.

The NHS (1948) accepted and developed the regional structure of the hospital service – with it came no new hospitals, no new or extra medical and nursing staff and no new administrators. It provided solely a new administrative framework. The NHS inherited the old hospitals, most of which are still functioning with adaptations, and few new hospitals have been built in the UK since 1948.

The hospital service as a separate part of the NHS has

its own highly trained specialist medical and nursing staff, and the administration follows a common pattern, each hospital being divided into a number of clinical departments with specialised beds under the clinical control of the consultant-in-charge of that department.

Under the NHS the Department of Health has the direct responsibility for the provision, on a national basis, of all hospital and specialist services, including those for mental disorders (with the exception of a very small number of private nursing homes and hospitals). In Scotland the Secretary of State for Scotland is the responsible Minister.

These services are organised regionally, the UK being divided into twenty Hospital Regions, each centred on a city with a university medical school. The Regional Hospital Boards (RHB) are responsible for the general planning and co-ordination of the hospital services in their respective regions, and they decide the major issues of policy, leaving day-to-day administration of the hospitals to local Hospital Management Committees.

The members of the Regional Hospital Boards are appointed by the Department of Health for a period of three years, and they are selected as representative of a cross-section of the whole community. All appointments are honorary and unpaid. The Minister also appoints the chairman of the RHB who, with the senior administrative medical officer of the Board, are key persons.

Hospital Management Committees (HMC), of which there are 400, act as agents of the RHB in day-to-day administration of a group of local hospitals. These have more routine responsibilities and are not concerned with major policy decisions, leaving these to the Regional Board. The members of these committees are appointed by the parent Board and reflect the special structure of the communities concerned, including not only physicians but members of local authorities, trade unionists and other members of the general public.

Each individual hospital, of which there are some 3,000, is administered by its own committee with a non-medical administrator–secretary.

In England and Wales the Teaching Hospitals are outside the authority of the Regional Boards and retain their own governing bodies. The Department of Health, however, retains responsibility for providing the clinical facilities, leaving to the universities the responsibility for provision of teaching.

There is, therefore, in the hospital system of the UK a flow of responsibilites from the Department of Health down to the individual hospital. Finance influences the whole system. It is through the Department of Health that the Regional Board receives its monies and in its turn allocates proportionate shares to the Hospital Management Committees.

TYPES OF HOSPITAL

The NHS has integrated the hospitals completely, and there is no distinction between the old voluntary and municipal hospitals.

The District Hospitals are of all sizes, and they act as community hospitals providing the first level of general hospital care. Including general surgical, medical, gynaecological, ear, nose and throat, and paediatric departments, they also provide out-patient specialist facilities for ambulatory patients in skin, psychiatric, eye, physical medicine and orthopaedic specialities.

The hospitals work closely together, and many specialists are on the staffs of more than one. Patients can be transferred easily from one hospital to another. Sub-regional specialities such as geriatric, eye, orthopaedic, infectious disease, psychiatric and accident units are located at one or other of the hospitals in a Hospital Management committee's district. The population served by an HMC averages 125,000, with ranges from nearly half a million to 50,000.

In each Regional Board's area there will be a number of regional specialist centres based on a large district hospital or in a separate hospital. These include units for neurosurgery and neurology, chest surgery and medicine, open-heart and vascular surgery, plastic surgery, the treatment of spinal injuries, rheumatic disease and others.

They act as centres to which patients may be referred either by general practitioners or by other hospital specialists. There is a good and easy flow of patients between these regional centres and district hospitals. Many of the specialists from the regional centres attend district hospitals for consulting sessions in the out-patient departments.

There are still many special hospitals for specific disorders such as mental illness, chest illness, obstetrics, geriatrics, infectious diseases, urology and others, but they are relics of the past. The present trend is to group all these specialities in a single large district hospital.

Teaching hospitals serve special functions. Most teaching hospitals are concerned primarily with undergraduate education; all undertake some postgraduate training for specialists but few engage widely in more general postgraduate training. Continuing education for general practitioners and general specialists is carried out at District Hospital Postgraduate Medical Centres, and of these there is approximately one in each Hospital Management Committee's area. The undergraduate and postgraduate teaching hospitals, in addition to their educational functions, also house many regional specialist centres and they include on their staffs some of the most eminent physicians in the land.

PARTICULAR ASPECTS OF IN-PATIENT CARE IN THE UNITED KINGDOM'S HOSPITALS

Beds in British hospitals tend to be arranged in large wards according to specialities. There are separate medical, surgical, gynaecological, eye, ENT, orthopaedic, paediatric and other wards in the larger hospitals. It has been customary for each specialist on the staff of the hospital to be allocated a set number of beds for his use and this has led to problems in efficient management and administration.

Patients are admitted to hospital either as emergencies through general practitioners, from the hospital's accident and emergency unit or from the 'waiting list'. This 'list' comprises patients who have been seen by specialists in their out-patient (ambulatory) clinics and whom they have recommended for admission. They are placed on a list and are admitted in rotation or according to the urgency of their medical needs and priorities. The length of time that a patient may have to wait depends on the hospital, the specialist and the condition requiring admission. Whilst patients with urgent and semi-urgent conditions such as neoplasms, peptic ulcers or those requiring special investigations may be admitted within one or two weeks, those with non-urgent conditions such as enlarged tonsils and adenoids, varicose veins, hernia, hallux valgus, haemorrhoids or vaginal prolapse may have to wait up to a year.

The proportion of patients attending an out-patient department who are subsequently admitted to hospital is between 15 and 25 per cent (*Problems and Progress in Medical Care*, Editor G. McLachlan, London, 1966).

A feature of the NHS is the domiciliary consultation scheme whereby a general practitioner may call out a specialist in consultation in the patient's own home, if he considers that patient too ill to attend the out-patient department and who might not require urgent admission to hospital. The specialist receives a fee from the NHS for such a consultation. Up to 200 such consultations may be carried out in any year, by any specialist. Geriatricians, psychiatrists and general medicine specialists receive the highest number of such calls, but the mean annual figure for domiciliary consultations is only 40 for each specialist in the NHS.

Certain district hospitals have recently been designated as local postgraduate medical centres for the continuing education of junior hospital staff and general practitioners, and these are administered through a national scheme with appointed regional deans and local clinical tutors.

PLANNING

Nationalisation of hospitals under the NHS made forward planning of all medical services a possibility, but it still tends to be piecemeal and unco-ordinated. Hospital services are planned without much relation to public health and general practice developments. The main trends are to set up larger district general hospital complexes of 1,000 or more beds, for the development of regional specialist centres, for the gradual run-down and closure of small units and for the incorporation of special hospitals, for mental diseases and others, into the general local hospital structure. The implementation of these and other planning policies has been through the Regional Hospital Board, and many have their own operational units involved in forward planning and continuing assessment of current work.

General Practice

Apart from a few exceptions, in rural areas and some special situations, general practitioners have been virtually excluded from the in-patients work in hospital. There are no real facilities for most general practitioners to admit and care for their own patients, nor are there any incentives for such work. General practitioners are remunerated by capitation fees and there are no provisions for fees for hospital care provided by the general practitioner. In those few hospitals where general practitioners can care for their own patients they receive no extra fees but rather a nominal honorarium. Approximately 2 per cent of all the UK hospital beds are available for the direct use of general practitioners, but even these tend to be used in an ineffectual way and the average annual daily occupancy rate is only 69 per cent for GP beds, compared with 85 per cent for the whole hospital system.

Hospitals provide diagnostic facilities for local general practitioners and some practitioners assist in the work of out-patient departments as 'clinical assistants' for which they receive a salary. Contacts between general practitioners and hospitals are through regular channels of communication in the course of management of their patients and through personal contact at professional meetings and domiciliary consultations.

Public Health Services

Relations between hospitals and local public health services exist at formal levels for public health purposes, but there is no sharing of staff and the Medical Officer of Health has no recognised role in the hospital service.

RESOURCES AND UTILISATION

In 1966 there were 9.6 hospital beds per 1,000 population in the United Kingdom. This rate has fallen since 1950 largely because of the reduction in the numbers of beds for mental diseases. (Table 28.)

TABLE 28

Hospital beds per 1,000 in England and Wales

	1950	1955	1960	1965	1966
General hospital beds per 1,000	4·6	5·1	5·4	5·3	5·3
Psychiatric beds per 1,000	5·3	5·1	4·6	4·1	4·0
Tuberculosis (and other chest diseases) beds per 1,000	0·6	0·5	0·4	0·3	0·3
TOTAL HOSPITAL BEDS PER 1,000	10·5	10·7	10·4	9·7	9·6

(Sources: Annual Reports of the Ministry of Health.)

These hospital beds were subdivided into specialities as shown in Table 29.

TABLE 29

Hospital beds per 1,000 in England and Wales in specialities for 1966

Speciality	Hospital beds per 1,000
Medical	
General medicine	0·7
Paediatrics	0·15
TB and other chest conditions	0·3
Infectious diseases	0·10
Neurology	0·03
Skin and VD	0·05
Others	0·07
Total	1·4
Surgical	
General surgery	0·7
ENT	0·13
Ophthalmology	0·10
Others	0·57
Total	1·5
Obstetrics	0·36
Gynaecology	0·20
Psychiatry	4·0
Geriatrics	0·65
Chronic sick	0·55
Others	0·94
TOTAL	9·6

(Source: Annual Report of Ministry of Health for 1966.)

In 1966, 10.5 per cent of all UK subjects were admitted to hospital on one or more occasion, and since 1956 the proportions admitted have increased, and the durations of stay have gradually decreased. (Table 30.)

TABLE 30

Bed-stay and admission rate (England and Wales)

	1956	1960	1964	1966
Total hospital admissions per 1,000	89	90	100*	105†
Average length of stay (days)	17·6	15·0	13·0	12·3

* Includes 5 per 1,000 in mental hospitals.
† Includes 6 per 1,000 in mental hospitals.

(Source: Annual Reports of Ministry of Health.)

In 1966 there were half a million patients in the UK waiting to be admitted to hospital. Surgical conditions accounted for 77 per cent of these and gynaecological conditions for a further 15 per cent. There was virtually no delay in admitting medical and other non-surgical conditions.

There are 19 consultant specialists in the UK, per 100,000 population, and 20 junior doctors per 100,000 working in support. Expressed in rates per 100 hospital beds, there were 5 physicians 50 nurses and 6 paramedical auxiliaries for every 100 hospital beds in 1966.

There is no special system of quality control in UK hospitals, reliance is placed on professional hospital committees and on the opinions of patients and their relatives.

TRENDS

The hospitals of the United Kingdom are admitting more patients for shorter stays. To increase efficiency and improve services larger general hospital units are being created, whilst smaller hospitals and those for special diseases are being closed. Attempts are also being made for the hospitals to play a greater role in community health.

Direct Comparisons of Hospital Care in the Three Countries

In the USA the hospital occupies the pre-eminent position

in medical care. The rate of hospitalisation is increasing steadily and is now at 15 per cent of the population each year, but in addition to this the ways in which it is being used for very short stay diagnostic admissions, encouraged by the terms and conditions of pre-paid insurance schemes, suggests that this rate of use will increase even more rapidly as a result of the new Medicare and Medicaid schemes.

In the USSR the hospital is a part of the Soviet system of medical care. The polyclinic, public health and the other community services have all been evolved and developed in step with hospital services, but in spite of this the hospitals with their own separate staffs, appear separated from any real involvement in community care and responsibilities.

The very high rate of hospitalisation of 20 per cent of the population per year, which is to be increased to 24 per cent in the future, implies a different use of the hospital from that in other systems. Surveys have found that one-third of Soviet citizens in medical and surgical wards were there needlessly and the custom of 'prophylactic' admissions to avoid possible complications in vulnerable persons has not been supported by any published investigations.

The hospital in the UK occupies a middle place between what one might call the short, sharp and rather quixotic use of hospitals in the USA and the more ponderous and extended use in the USSR. With its integrated out-patient department the British hospital is better able to screen those requiring admission and to carry out many investigations and procedures normally undertaken inside a US hospital. The Soviet polyclinic does not quite fulfil the functions of the British hospital out-patient department, for the polyclinic specialists do not work in a hospital. They are less experienced in hospital-type diseases than are British specialists who all work in hospital as well as in out-patient clinics. Consequently many Soviet citizens are being admitted for diagnostic and other purposes because of this separation of polyclinic and hospital medical staffs.

IN-PATIENT CARE

The extent of hospitalisation ranges from 20 per cent of the population in the USSR to 15 per cent in the USA to 10 per cent in the UK.

The types of cases admitted to hospital differ. Those in the UK are there more for technical and therapeutic purposes, than for a diagnostic work-up which is carried out in the out-patient departments. Patients in the wards of British hospitals appear generally to be more ill than those in hospitals in the USA and the USSR perhaps because of the differences in selection for admission. Many of those who are in hospitals in the USSR and the USA would be treated in their homes by British general practitioners.

SPECIALIST CARE FOR AMBULATORY PATIENTS

Soviet hospitals are not involved in care for ambulatory patients, such care being carried out in polyclinics. In the USA with its system of private, fee-for-service practice, ambulatory and specialist care is carried out in the physicians' own consulting rooms or private clinics. Some community hospitals do provide out-patient clinics for medical indigents who cannot afford private care.

In the UK the specialist service for the ambulatory is provided in the hospital out-patient department and some 15 per cent of the population are referred to these departments each year.

COMMUNITY RESPONSIBILITIES

Whilst it is clear that the hospital is but a part of the total health services with responsibilities to the community outside, it is only in the USSR that hospitals really are involved in health education and preventive care.

STRUCTURE AND ADMINISTRATION

History and traditions have influenced the structural patterns of the hospital systems.

In the USSR a young system has attempted to integrate hospitals with other services at local and national levels, and from the centre to the periphery there is a clear and understandable pattern of administration, supported by a system of norms and standards that underlies operational research and future planning. Based on the geographical and territorial divisions of republic, region and district, there is an accepted hierarchical structure of administrative roles and responsibilities. In the Soviet system there are no problems concerning controls, power and orders. Levels of authority are understood clearly and orders and directions readily accepted.

In the UK a new scheme, the NHS has been superimposed on a little-altered system with traditional separation of hospital from the community services. Whilst it has led to considerable improvements in regionalisation of hospital services with a more rational approach to utilisation, there have been few developments to integrate the three parts of the service even at local levels. The administrative structure of the NHS shows a paradox of ministerial power and impotence.

In theory the Secretary of State for the Department of Health has the overriding responsibility for all major and other policy matters; in fact he has to deal and negotiate with a highly independent, conservative and tradition-bound profession. The administration of hospitals in the UK is shared by professional lay (non-medical) administrators, by amateur lay committee members appointed in various ways and by physicians who spend some of their time on various committees in a voluntary and unpaid capacity.

In the USA the characteristic is that of independence of action. Hospitals have been allowed to develop according to local pressures and wealth, with scant attention to real medical and social needs.

Hospitals in many parts of the USA are in active competition for fee-paying patients to fill their beds, and only recently have any realistic attempts been started to plan hospital services in a collaborative and rational fashion.

Hospital administration is a highly developed profession. Hospital administrators may be medically qualified, university graduates in medical administration or businessmen who have been attracted to the field of hospital management. Much of their time is taken up with finance and in raising money to provide their services.

PROBLEMS OF RURAL AREAS

Great problems arise in providing hospital services to scattered rural communities in the USSR and the USA.

In the USSR accessible hospital services have been provided by the system of small *'uchastok'* rural hospitals (15–100 beds), each combined with a polyclinic and associated feldsher–midwife posts. The problem of medical staffing has been dealt with by directing young physicians to rural areas for up to three years after qualification.

In the USA no set pattern has emerged. It has been left largely to the outlying communities themselves to attract physicians to their localities to staff small rural hospitals which they build and run themselves.

RESOURCES AND UTILISATION

Table 31 shows the present state of hospital resources and data on utilisation.

TABLE 31

Comparison of hospital resources and utilisation data

	USSR	USA	UK
Hospitals beds per 1,000 population			
General	8·67	4·9	5·6
Psychiatric	0·93	4·0	4·0
TOTAL	9·6	8·9	9·6
Staff per 100 beds			
Physicians	9	10*	5
Nurses	38	59	56
Utilisation			
Admissions per 100	20%	15%	10%
Average length of stay per patient (days)	15–16	9–10	12–13

* Estimated – most are part-time.

Although the total rates of hospital beds per 1,000 population are comparable there is a very great difference in the proportions for psychiatric and non-psychiatric conditions. Whereas the rates for psychiatric beds are the same in the USA and the UK, they are four times greater than the rate in the USSR. Even with the proposed doubling of beds for mental illness in the USSR the rate will still be only one-half of the USA and the UK.

The explanation is elusive. It may be that there is a real smaller need for such beds in the USSR because there is less mental illness, or perhaps there is active discouragement of such illnesses and little readiness to provide hospital facilities (see also Chapter 10). Because there are so few beds for mental illnesses there are proportionately many more beds available for non-psychiatric conditions. This may well explain the high level of utilisation, i.e. 20 per cent admitted each year and the longer average stay in hospital.

When the rates of staff per 100 beds are considered they are comparable in the USSR and the UK because in both nations the staff are full-time hospital employees, but in the USA most physicians work part-time only on hospital duties. There are twice as many physicians per 100 beds in the USSR than in the UK, but fewer nurses.

The most striking difference between the three nations is in the open-staffing policy in the USA where most local physicians, including doctors-of-first-contact, have access to hospital beds. That is, they are all on the staff of the hospital and are free to admit and treat patients under their care. The prevailing system of remuneration, by fees for services, encourages such admissions, and it inevitably results in physicians caring for a whole range of complex conditions, often outside their own speciality and beyond their experience.

Remuneration of hospital staff in the USSR is by salary according to seniority, experience and merit, and according to grades of speciality.

In the UK hospital care is the responsibility of specialists who are appointed by competitive selection, and they are paid either by a salary, according to seniority, or on a sessional basis, when they may also engage in private practice. There is also a system of 'merit awards' whereby many specialists receive extra annual remuneration according to an assessment by a special committee of senior physicians.

Comparison of the quality of the hospital services in the three nations is difficult because there are no ready, reliable and acceptable objective measures available.

Thus, if the criterion of availability and accessibility is considered, and it is certainly a justified measure of quality of medical care, then the USSR and the UK have reached a higher level of achievement than has the USA where the geographical, social and economic barriers still exist.

The quality of medical buildings such as hospitals, clinics and physicians' rooms is unquestionably the highest in the

USA, there are many old but functional units in the UK, and there are many new 'instant' hospitals and polyclinics in the USSR.

Essential equipment is available in all three nations. There is also much equipment with an obvious local flavour and rather questionable usefulness such as the hydrotherapy units in the USSR, the computers in the USA and the physical medicine departments in the UK.

The quality of staff is impossible to measure. In the USSR there are no apparent shortages of nurses or doctors, and it is not possible to fault their work. In the USA the staff of many hospitals is part-time and many physicians in charge of patients would seem to have a lack of experience in some of the rarer conditions which they seek to treat. However, where there is a satisfactory staffing of full-time specialists in the hospital and ready referral between the specialists and specialoids, then the service combines the ideals of continuing personal care and specialist expertise. In the UK the quality of all hospital specialists is high – because of the long training and the competition for appointments.

As the ultimate index of quality the *results of care* appear comparable overall in the three nations. There seem to be no great differences in the end results of the common hospital diseases. The inevitable failures are those inherent in the diseases rather than in the quality of care.

Personal Evaluation

A key question in medical care is where and how should the modern hospital fit into any system? Hospital services are the most expensive and the most expert section in medical care and it is essential that they be used economically and for maximum effect and benefits. Even a superficial examination of hospital services reveals gross inefficiencies, wastages and uncertainties over roles and functions. Comparisons between the USSR, the USA and the UK show considerable differences in all parts and levels of the hospital services and these differences raise important questions on the effective use of hospitals.

The ideal form in which medical care should be organised is not yet apparent, but it is clear that the following principles must be incorporated:

Hospitals

An integrated system of medical care requires the bringing together of the various parts, i.e. hospitals, first-contact and specialist ambulatory care and public health services. The hospital service cannot function effectively without such integration.

Planning for hospital services requires definition of certain levels of care and responsibility. These levels must be related to population size and geography.

Suitable levels would be:

1. National
2. Republic or State
3. Regional
4. District
5. Neighbourhood (2,000–50,000).

At each level, responsibility for managerial administration and organisation should rest with individuals who must be supported by committees and other statutory bodies.

Although there are some facts and data available on the ways in which hospitals are being used, there is need for more detailed information supported by planned operational experiments designed to test certain hypotheses, as at present available data suggests misuse and over-use of hospital facilities in all three countries.

Estimates for the future will have to take account of new methods and techniques which may on the one hand require more physicians and nurses, but which on the other hand may save manpower resources by more efficiency.

There are difficulties on both scores. The various indices of measuring quality of care in hospitals are not satisfactory, nor is it easy to use them to compare the quality of individual hospitals let alone national hospital systems, and further work is necessary to arrive at more readily accessible criteria of the quality of hospital care.

Chapter 7
Preventive Aspects of Medical Care

'Prevention' of disease and maintenance of sound health are the ultimate goals of good medical care.

The control of the major diseases that were associated with poverty, neglect, insanitation and an inadequacy of medical resources, has however changed the pace of medical care, and we are now faced with those related to modern affluent societies, namely the care of an ageing population with degenerative disorders such as cancer, strokes, high blood pressure, coronary heart disease, chronic chest ailments, mental disorders and their related social problems.

Unquestionably it was far easier to prevent the old-type diseases than those associated with modern living, and it is not certain yet how successful are the modern techniques of prevention.

Preventive Medicine in the USSR

'Prevention' is one of the major principles on which Soviet medical care is based.

The preventive approach has permeated every level of care and all practising physicians are involved in applying general and specific measures that are designed to prevent the development and progression of disease. Side by side with the more general achievements such as the control of poverty, improvements in hygiene and sanitation, education and the provision of adequate medical and paramedical resources, there have been developed specific systems and methods directed to prevention. The major efforts in this direction have been towards the 'dispensarisation scheme'.

This scheme, so called because originally it was based on 'dispensaries', is the chief method of planned preventive care in the USSR, its *aims* are:

1. Early diagnosis of clinical and social disorders by means of regular screening and examinations of the population.
2. Definition and delineation of vulnerable groups and individuals as well as the diagnosis of specific diseases.
3. The correction of underlying predisposing causes, social as well as medical and the early treatment of medical conditions.
4. The follow-up of vulnerable groups. (These tend to be persons diagnosed as suffering from certain specified diseases.)
5. Rehabilitation.

At present the 'dispensarisation' scheme is confined to certain groups of the population such as children, adolescents, workers in some hazardous occupations, expectant mothers, sportsmen and sportswomen and any persons known to be suffering from chronic conditions. These groups cover 83 million out of 230 million Soviet citizens who are examined each year under the scheme.

One reason given for increasing the numbers of physicians and resources in the USSR is that it is planned that ultimately every Soviet citizen should be covered by the 'dispensarisation' scheme and examined each year.

The whole scheme is organised and administered through, and in co-operation with, the local public health unit, and the polyclinics. The polyclinics are responsible for the selection and follow-up, and the public health service is brought in to correct, where possible, any social factors discovered. The selection of persons for this medical supervision is part of the work of the polyclinic organisation, and registers are compiled, with patients being notified when they are required for examination or follow-up. Any examination and screening is carried out first by the individual's own local paediatrician or therapist (the first-contact-physicians), and if any abnormalities are discovered then one of the polyclinic specialists is brought in to help in diagnosis and assessment. A set routine of examination, investigation, recording, grading and procedure is followed for each specified group.

The assessment of the person's problems is the next step and this naturally involves a social as well as a medical diagnosis. Certain specific conditions, once diagnosed, are recognised as requiring special management and follow-up and these include peptic ulcer, hypertension, coronary heart disease and other forms of heart disease, glaucoma, obesity, chronic bronchitis and asthma, tuberculosis, cancer, strokes and many others. The type of 'social factor' that is assessed includes, amongst others, the patient's housing conditions, work-record and satisfaction, and their marital state and harmony.

Having made a diagnosis and assessment, appropriate therapy and management are arranged for specific medical conditions and follow-up is mandatory to ensure progress. Housing problems, for example, may be referred to the local public health service for further action, and this organisation has powers to instruct local housing authorities to rehouse families who are living in poor conditions. In addition to a personal programme of care, the patient may also be invited, with his relatives, to attend for group therapy. Such group therapy is used particularly in the care of persons with peptic ulcers, hypertension, obesity and mental illness. Rehabilitation and physical therapy may be provided, convalescent holidays arranged and special diets supplied.

The 'dispensarisation' scheme accounts for a sizeable proportion of the physicians' work, and between 10 and 20 per cent of the 'local' therapist's time is spent on routine examinations, whilst this proportion is up to 50–60 per cent of the time of the paediatrician. Although attempts have been made to evaluate the success of all these schemes, there have, as yet, been no reports of critical assessments published.

Great emphasis has been placed on health education in the Soviet system of medical care, so that the individual may exercise his own responsibilities in maintaining his health and fitness. Major efforts have been made at national and local levels to encourage public participation in courses and lectures and in the dissemination of knowledge on health through publications, radio and television. It is estimated for example, that 45 million Soviet citizens, or almost half the working adult population, have passed through special health education courses that included personal health maintenance, hygiene, public health measures and sanitation, the organisation of medical services, and first-aid. Locally, health education is organised through the polyclinics, with a special social worker engaged in arranging lectures and demonstrations for the public, and every physician is expected to devote 4–5 hours of each week to this form of health education.

Health is considered to be the personal responsibility of each individual and there are excellent facilities for sport, exercise and other leisure pursuits. There are also a large number of spas and convalescent and holiday homes for those requiring rehabilitation.

In addition to the principle of individual self-help, there are 'health volunteer activists', who, having taken further training in public health maintenance, are given some powers and responsibilities for supervision of public health measures, sanitation and hygiene in their own immediate localities and it is estimated that there is one health 'activist' to about ten dwellings. These health 'activists' undertake regular hygienic inspections and supervision and they co-operate with polyclinics in organising the dispensarisation scheme, particularly in reminding and encouraging persons to attend for follow-up examinations.

Preventive Medicine in the USA

The principles of prevention and health maintenance have been accepted and developed over the years in the USA but it has not been possible to apply the full facilities and benefits to the whole population. Whilst primary measures such as better hygiene and sanitation and secondary measures such as immunisation have been available to all, steps to encourage early diagnosis and treatment through the 'medical check-up' have been available only to certain social, economic and occupational groups.

THE 'MEDICAL CHECK-UP'

The regular annual medical check-up has developed as a specific preventive exercise, that has been supported strongly by the medical profession and generally accepted by the public. Nevertheless it is confined to those who are either able to pay for it, or to those who are covered by various insurance or occupational schemes. Although there is no reliable data it is probable that about 20 per cent of the US public (including children) are covered by such a scheme. Those who are covered are chiefly the very young and the middle-aged – the young through well-baby care schemes and the middle-aged through publicity and health education directed at them as 'vulnerables'. The procedure of the medical check-up has been encouraged strongly by the medical profession, and it now takes up a considerable proportion of the work of the internists and the paediatrician and it also represents a considerable source of income.

The techniques comprise an opportunity to take a history, a physical examination and a battery of tests, but no satisfactory evaluations of the medical check-up scheme have been made. Although many reports suggest an appreciable rate of abnormalities (in up to one-third of those examined), the real significance of these findings is still uncertain. Thus, it is not yet clear whether early diagnosis makes any difference to the final outcome in persons found to be suffering from disorders such as diabetes, hypertension, and even cancer of the breast, cervix and lung.

Preventive Medicine in the UK

In the United Kingdom there has been slow acceptance of the idea of such preventive procedures as general pre-symptomatic screening. Primary and secondary measures of prevention, namely, eradication of causes and widespread immunisation have been followed actively and there is now a high level of artificial immunity in the population against poliomyelitis, diphtheria, whooping cough, tetanus and smallpox. The 'medical check-up', however, and various more specific screening procedures designed for wholesale and routine use, such as cervical cytology and checks for high blood pressure, glaucoma, diabetes and anaemia, are still being critically evaluated. It has been the policy of the Department of Health to support and to encourage cervical cytology, miniature mass radiography of the chest and tests for phenylketonuria, but no national policy has been decided yet on more general screening.

Preventive care under the NHS is shared by all three divisions of the service with general practitioners involved in antenatal care, child welfare, immunisation and cervical cytology programmes; local authority services providing the same facilities as do general practitioners (because not all general practitioners have agreed to participate in such activities); and hospitals through the Regional Hospital Boards remaining responsible for miniature mass radiography services, for much antenatal care of women delivered in the hospital and for specific procedures such as cervical cytology and other diagnostic procedures.

Comparison of the Preventive Services

In all three nations there is general acceptance that prevention is a desirable ideal and worthy of great effort in order to achieve success, but great differences exist in the extent of acceptance of procedures that inevitably require a considerable expenditure of resources that are already under strain.

In the USSR enthusiastic acceptance of the principle of prevention has created a special scheme which embodies not only early diagnosis, but also measures to define and correct social as well as medical causes of disease and disorder, and to ensure the follow-up and supervision of vulnerable groups in order to prevent breakdown and recurrence in the future.

In the USA in addition to the standard procedures of public health hygiene and the immunisation of children, emphasis has been placed on the 'medical check-up' involving regular (annual if possible) medical examination accompanied by a battery of tests and investigations in order to detect early signs of disease. At present such services are confined to those who are able to afford to pay for the services, but in the future with the development of automated techniques of investigation it is hoped to extend such examinations to an increasing proportion of the public.

In the UK, due to its traditional and rather conservative beliefs, mass screening has not been introduced generally on a wide scale. Individual practitioners are free to carry out procedures that they consider necessary and useful but there are no financial incentives for regular check-ups. There are however some financial inducements for general practitioners to carry out immunisation and cervical cytology the physicians who carry out such services for their patients are able to claim and receive extra fees.

A Personal Evaluation

The present situation of the preventive aspects of medical care is in varying degrees of progression in the three nations and in view of the differences of opinion and procedure, it seems that no major policy decisions involving deployment and use of considerable resources should be made until there is more proof available as to their merits.

Whilst there is general acceptance, based on definite proof, of well-established immunisation and hygienic procedures, there is no such reliable proof of the efficacy and usefulness of time-consuming measures like regular check-ups, screening, examination and the routine investigation of large sections of the population.

Not only is there no proof that many of so-called 'significant' abnormalities detected at such screening are really abnormal, but there is also no proof that early diagnosis and subsequent treatment in the pre-symptomatic phase alters the final outcome. (*Screening in Medical Care*, Mc-Lachlan, G. (ed.), London (1968) and *Early Diagnosis* (1968–9), published by Office of Health Economics London.) A compromise therefore is necessary between over-enthusiasm and over-ready acceptance of fashionable trends, and the implementation of well-established preventive measures. Should final proof be forthcoming that regular screening methods are worth while then the 'dispensarisation' scheme evolved in the USSR provides a good example for the way in which a comprehensive programme could be developed.

Chapter 8
Public Health and Social Services

Public health services are having to meet new and changing needs in the modern developed society. In comparison with modern needs, those of the past, such as providing clean water and food, sanitation and control of epidemics, appear straightforward to those of today. Modern public health services are now tackling the challenges of prevention and alleviation of disorders of degeneration and ageing and they are endeavouring to educate their populations towards self-help and healthier living – the detrimental effects of the cigarette-smoking habit and the problems of its control are a particular modern example. They are concerned in providing services for the physically and mentally handicapped. They are involved in community care and welfare for certain recognised vulnerable groups such as expectant mothers, children, the mentally sick, the tuberculous and the elderly, but the increasing frequency and diversity of social pathology in our modern society with conditions such as drug taking and alcoholism, adolescent delinquency, promiscuity and illegitimacy are creating new tasks for public health services. In some places the Medical Officer of Health is developing as an epidemiologist, administrator, and planner of medical care.

Public Health Services in the USSR

In Soviet Russia these services are based on a series of 'Sanitary and Epidemiological Stations' (*Sanepids*), which are staffed by specialist physicians, 'hygienists'. They receive a special training from the undergraduate period onwards to fit them for their professional career as Medical Officers of Health in the public health service. There is at least one general public health unit in every district and these are linked with more specialised regional units. Usually based on a district, the typical soviet 'health unit' has, on average, a population of 50,000 to supervise and care for, and there are some 5,000 such units in the USSR with a staff of 40;000 physicians (7–8 per cent of all medical manpower).

The role of the public health service is both supervisory, in checking and maintaining levels of hygiene and sanitation in their area, and organisational, in taking positive steps to improve the working and living conditions of the people.

The control and eradication of infectious diseases is brought about through a system of notification and morbidity recording at the polyclinics. Following receipt of notification of infectious disease the public health physicians employ wide powers for compulsory hospitalisation, the quarantine of infected persons, and for the disinfection of premises. The local public health unit is also responsible for ensuring high levels of protection against infectious diseases through general hygienic and sanitary measures and through a mass immunisation programme against accepted diseases that include smallpox, diphtheria, tetanus, whooping cough, poliomyelitis, tuberculosis and measles.

These units work closely with local polyclinics and hospitals and all three are under the control of a single chief physician of the District to whom the hygienist in charge of the public health services is responsible. A section of the service is responsible for ensuring what one might call 'optimal environmental conditions' for the physical and emotional development of children. This is done through co-operation with the paediatricians of the polyclinic and also through supervision of the building and maintenance of local crèches, nurseries, kindergartens and schools. More generally, the public health units bear the responsibilility for ensuring a balanced diet and safe foods, for the provision and maintenance of amenities for 'rest' and facilities for exercise, leisure and recreation.

As noted in Chapter 7, the unit is also much involved in the organisation of the 'dispensarisation' scheme, and health education.

The organisation of the public health service is based on the standard territorial structure of the USSR with departments at all levels from the Ministry and Republic, through the region to the district and down to the feldshers who carry out sanitary and epidemiological work in outlying rural areas.

In a typical district unit there are three main departments, hygiene, epidemiological control and administration, and the work of each department is based on the 'locality' principle whereby physicians and paramedical assistants are given responsibilities for a particular territorial district. Each unit has its own laboratories specialising in public health work and co-operating closely with those in hospitals and polyclinics. It is the central co-ordinating unit for operational studies and the analysing of data that is sent to it continually from the local hospitals and polyclinics. It is also in close contact with many local non-medical organisations such as trade unions, industrial units, Red Cross and Red Crescent organisations, public health volunteers and elected representatives of the public, and to all these it acts as an advisor in public health matters.

The department of hygiene will deal with the more general public health matters, which include communal hygiene, housing and schools, etc.: with occupational and industrial health involving the supervision of industrial premises, new technical processes, noise, radioactivity and the health of workers; food hygiene, involving the supervision of the whole food industry from manufacture, through distribution to retail; and with the health of children and adolescents, their development, school buildings, hygiene and diet.

The epidemiology department is concerned with the control of epidemics and prevention of infectious disease through notification, planning of local preventive measures, supervision and advice to local hospitals and polyclinics and the assay of the efficacy of antibiotics and similar drugs in the control of epidemic foci.

The administrative department not only receives for analysis all the polyclinic and hospital data that relate to the nature and the volume of their work, but also carries out a 'health-census' every five years in an attempt to assess the state of health, morbidity, social status and the use of the available resources in its area.

The 'Hygienist', or Medical Officer of Health has a high status in the Soviet medical hierarchy. He is recognised as a specialist on account of his special undergraduate and postgraduate training and he has considerable statutory powers of direction over all other physicians and medical establishments.

He is involved actively in the forward planning of all medical services in the district and carries out quality assessments of the various medical services.

Public Health Services in the USA

In America these services exist as a separate branch from the clinical services, but they share many points of contact. Because of the system of free enterprise and individual responsibilities for meeting the costs of medical care, the provisions of care for the medical indigents, who cannot afford to meet the costs of private care, have become the responsibility of the State and government authorities through the public health service. Many hospitals and health clinics therefore are provided and administered through the public health service in the USA.

With a national structure of Federal, State and local levels of administration, the public health services follow the same pattern. At the Federal level is the US Public Health Service, which is a part of the Health, Education and Welfare Department, and this service exists chiefly as a central consultative research and co-ordinating body, with little involvement in local public health activities. Individual States have considerable automony in matters of public health, with each State having its own Board of Health with two main departments of health and public welfare. The State Department of Health deals with public health and sanitation, control of communicable diseases, local community nursing services and special programmes relating to maternal and child health, dental care and mental health. There is also a special division administering the State hospital services. The State Department of Public Welfare has divisions responsible for the welfare of handicapped and deprived children, for community care of mental illness, tuberculosis and various social disorders. Public financial assistance, including old age assistance, aid to dependent children and the disabled and general relief are all administered through this department.

Locally, cities, municipalities and counties are often direct providers of hospitals, institutions for the aged and chronic sick and welfare facilities of various types.

Under the direction of the City (or County) Medical Officer of Health, extensive personal health services may be provided for various needy groups of the population, but each locality has its own schemes and interests and there is no uniform system or scheme applicable to all areas.

It is not surprising therefore, with this diversity of responsibility that there is little evidence of co-ordination and collaboration between the public health and local government services and the non-government medical services who provide private medical care.

Public Health Services in the UK

The public health service is one of the distinct divisions of the NHS, the other two being general practice and the hospital service. It is independent and autonomous, as part of the local government system, and it is administered by the county and borough councils through health committees with the Medical Officer of Health as a full-time employee in charge. The Department of Health has indirect responsibilities for local public health services and it formulates national policies but is not concerned with local details. Control of such policies is exercised through large grants that are paid from the Department to local authorities for health and social welfare purposes.

The Local Authority, through its public health department, provides institutional welfare nursing care for the chronic sick and aged, and organises and administers the ambulance services, and is involved with personal care services.

The Medical Officer of Health has a number of Assistant Medical Officers in the medical complement, each with certain fields of responsibility, and other staff include home nurses, district midwives and health visitors (public health nurses). There are also various general and special social workers involved in the care of the handicapped, the aged, children and expectant mothers, mental illnesses, tuberculosis, social problems and health education.

There have been signs recently that much better co-ordination in their fields of work, – between the public health authorities and the doctor-of-first-contact – is occurring. In many areas health visitors, home nurses and midwives are being attached to general practices and 'health teams' of these workers are emerging as effective and viable units. General practitioners are also becoming enthusiastic about working from health centres, specially designed and staffed by such teams, which are in certain areas being built by the local authorities with grants from the Department of Health. Relations between public health services and hospitals are in general still on a formal and distant plane. There are exceptions, however, and examples in some areas of excellent co-operation are in the fields of mental health care, maternity and child welfare and care for the aged – in such areas all the general practice, public health and hospital services often work together closely and harmoniously.

The chief official in the local authority health department is the Medical Officer of Health and by statute he must be a fully qualified physician with a recognised postgraduate training and qualification in public health. In addition he is usually the chief official of the Welfare Department.

Direct Comparison of the Public Health Services

In the USSR the public health services are not concerned with the organisation of hospitals, nor very much with personal health care, which is the task of the polyclinics, but they are very much involved with general public health procedures and with the operational planning of all local medical care services.

In the USA because of the system of care that creates a large group of medical indigents who cannot afford private medical care, the local health authorities provide, through the public health services, hospital and personal health care in addition to the standard public health and welfare services.

In the UK links with the traditional past have not yet been severed and there is an interim situation where, in spite of a National Health Service, there is a considerable overlap and a duplicity of care in the field of personal medical care. This applies particularly to facilities for child welfare and for care of the socially and physically handicapped of all types.

Lack of full integration between public health and other medical services is evident particularly in the USA and the

M

UK, where separation, competition and antagonism are evident. In the USSR, however, integration has been achieved and efforts have been made to give the public health services new roles and opportunities that match the demands of modern medical care for the community.

A Personal Evaluation

The trend in all three nations is for the public health services to become less involved with personal care and hospital services, and more concerned with the general care of large populations involved in hygiene, sanitation and environment safety and with the social and welfare problems of special groups of the population. They are becoming more concerned also with the epidemiological aspect of all types of diseases and with operational aspects of planning and administering medical care as a whole.

If they are to be able to exercise their potentials there must, however, be closer collaboration between the public health services and other branches of medical care especially hospitals and first-contact services and ideally, all medical and social services in any area should be integrated into a single service – with a single medical director or administrator responsible for organisation and planning.

Chapter 9
Maternity and Child Care

A high quality of maternal and child care is the best foundation for the future of any nation and the standards of care in this field offer particularly useful indices on the social and medical progress, of any country.

Maternity Services in the USSR

The visitor to Soviet Russia is informed repeatedly that 'the children are our only privileged class' and that 'the future of the nation rests on the health of our children', and great importance is obviously placed on services for expectant mothers and young children in the USSR.

A nation-wide system exists for the care of the expectant mother that is freely available and accessible. The pattern and routine of antenatal care are acceptable to the public and it is part of the health educational process to ensure that everyone understands the importance of regular ante-natal care and knows the steps to be taken when pregnancy is suspected.

Expectant mothers receive considerable safeguards and protection from the State in the USSR. Working mothers receive four months' compulsory paid leave and up to one year's unpaid leave of absence if necessary, and their jobs are kept open. In employment they have equal rights and pay as men. Those who are not at work receive grants and other support if required during the pregnancy and postnatal period.

The forms and patterns of maternity services differ according to the type of area. In large city urban areas care is based on the Women's Consultation Centre (WCC) and maternity hospitals, whereas in smaller towns and rural areas it is provided through the general polyclinic in association with District or local hospitals. Wherever it is carried out the routine is the same, with frequent and regular antenatal attendances from the third month of pregnancy onwards, delivery in maternity hospital, and close supervision in the postnatal phase.

Antenatal Care

The diagnosis of pregnancy is made either by the patient's regular local therapist or gynaecologist at the polyclinic, or in large towns the woman may go direct to the WCC in the first instance. This Women's Clinic serves not only as the local centre for antenatal and postnatal care, but also provides care for all 'women's ailments', including gynaecology, birth control, screening for cervical cancer, legal abortions and general advice on matters such as marriage counselling, separation and divorce and maintenance for the deserted wife. There is, in addition to the medical, nursing and social worker staff, a legal adviser attached to all clinics to assist women with such problems. It may be sited in the grounds of a maternity hospital but many are situated in the community some distance from the hospital. These separate clinics in urban areas tend to have their own separate staff. The total population cared for by such organisations in an urban district ranges from 50,000 to 150,000 and a maternity hospital will be linked with a number of Women's Clinics. There are local obstetrician–gynaecologists who are given territorial neighbourhoods and are responsible for all expectant mothers in their area. Each of these obstetricians works with a number of nurses and midwives in organising the antenatal care for her patients, and regular attendances are made by the expectant mother from the third month onwards, as a rule 12–16 such attendances are made during the antenatal period. Psychoprophylaxis, on Pavlovian principles, is carried out as a routine and mothercraft classes are held and attended regularly. In the smaller towns the same pattern of care is provided at the local polyclinic and in rural areas antenatal care is carried out by the feldsher–midwife working in association with the obstetrician at the local hospital.

DELIVERY

Almost all confinements are conducted at maternity hospitals, and home deliveries are strongly discouraged although a few still occur in rural areas. Midwives undertake normal deliveries under the supervision of obstetricians. Operative interference is reduced to a minimum and much reliance is placed on 'natural' childbirth under psychoprophylaxis. There is one bed per 1,000 for maternity care and the average length of stay is 8–9 days.

All postnatal care, after discharge from hospital, is carried out at the Women's Clinic or polyclinic and the woman reports soon after discharge from hospital and finally before return to work, two months after the birth.

BIRTH CONTROL

The birth rate in the USSR is falling and is now (1968) reported to be 18·4 per 1,000. (It was 25 per 1,000 in 1958/59.) However, this figure conceals the fact that in the Russian Republic (European part of the USSR) the birth rates are lower, i.e. 15·8 per 1,000 and in Moscow it is only 11 per 1,000, and in Latvia 13·9 per 1,000, whereas in the central Asiatic parts of the USSR the rates are much higher, over 25 per 1,000. (*The Times* of London, 29 Feb. 1968.)

The reasons for the reduction of the birth rate in the larger cities of the USSR are said to be that wives are working and prefer to work rather than to look after children, and that housing facilities are poor for large families. The average size of a young family in Moscow is 1–2 children. This falling birth rate has led to a national policy of discouragement of birth control, although advice is available, if asked for, at the Women's Clinic. The methods used are chiefly mechanical check-barriers, advice on withdrawal, chemical spermicides and douches. Contraceptive pills have not yet been introduced on any scale.

LEGALISED ABORTION

Termination of pregnancy was re-legalised in the USSR in 1955, but it is not encouraged. Any woman may ask to have her pregnancy terminated before the twelfth week but she must consult an obstetrician at the Women's Clinic who is empowered to discourage her from the act, but who is not permitted by law to refuse to carry out an abortion. Unlike other forms of hospital treatment, which are free of charge, termination of pregnancy, unless for definite medical or social reasons, has to be paid for by the woman. According to K.H. Mehland (1966) (*World Medical Journal*, *13*, 84) the proportion of abortions to births in the USSR is 1 : 1, therefore it is estimated that there are 4–5 million legalised abortions annually. The rates for abortions are highest in large towns, the proportion of births to abortions being 1 : 1·5, low in rural parts of European Russia, 1 : 0·5 and lowest in Asiatic parts of rural USSR, 1 : 0·3.

QUALITATIVE INDICES OF MATERNITY CARE

The qualitative indices of maternity care in the USSR are shown in Table 32.

TABLE 32

Qualitative indices of maternity care in the USSR

Birth rate per 1,000	Maternal mortality per 100,000 births	Infant mortality per 1,000 births
18·4	32*	28

*For Ukraine in 1959 the rate was 49.
(Sources: *The Times*, 29 Feb. 1968. Communication to WHO seminar in 1967. WHO demographic records.)

CHILD CARE SERVICES

The care of children is supported at all levels and in all circumstances by the State. There are special money grants and other aids to mothers with large families (three or more children), to those who breast-feed their babies, and to unmarried mothers (who receive a grant until the child reaches the age of 12). A nursing mother who is at work is allowed time each day to feed her child at home or in the crèche and if the child is sick and is being treated at home the mother is allowed to look after her child without losing wages. If the child is admitted to hospital the mother can go with the child and will continue to receive her wages.

The care of Soviet children is carried out from polyclinics and children's hospitals, and in large cities these children's

clinics are usually separate and distinct from other polyclinics. Each children's polyclinic cares for 10,000–15,000
children up to the age of 15. (See also Chapter 4.)

In smaller towns the care of children may be carried out at
a general polyclinic but by a special and separate department
with its own staff.

Children's hospitals may exist also as separate units or
there may be a children's unit in a District or Regional
hospital with its own staff and organisation. A children's
hospital may have a polyclinic attached to it.

First-contact care for children is provided by the local
paediatrician from the polyclinic, who cares for 750–1,250
children up to 15 years of age, including 40–50 babies in
their first year of life. Each paediatrician has one or more
nurses working with her, and these nurses assist the physician
in the polyclinic, supervise well-child care and preventive
measures and visit children and mothers in their homes.
Associated with the paediatricians are a number of specialists
to whom children may be referred, and special arrangements
are made to care for vulnerable children under the 'dispensarisation' scheme. In rural areas it is the feldsher who provides the first medical contact, and she supervises normal
child care, preventive and health educational measures and
the treatment of children's minor ailments under the supervision of a paediatrician.

ROUTINE OF CHILD CARE

Great emphasis is placed on the preventive nature of the
work of the child care services and in fact the major proportion of their work is devoted to preventive measures rather
than to traditional curative therapy.

Care for the infant begins in the prenatal period with a
home visit by the local paediatrician and her nurse to the
expectant mother to ensure that all facilities will be available when she returns home after the delivery, and to dis-
cuss the arrangements for regular supervision at the polyclinic. By law the paediatrician and nurse must visit the
mother and infant at home within a few days of their return
from maternity hospital, usually on the 10th–14th days of
life, for general assessment and advice. During the first year
the nurse pays regular visits to the home and the infant also

attends the polyclinic monthly to be seen by the paediatrician. During these monthly attendances the child's development is assessed and a schedule of immunisation carried out. During the second year a normal child is seen every three months at the polyclinic; in the third year he is seen twice, and, thereafter, from 3–7 years, once a year.

A special pre-school examination (at 6–7 years) is carried out jointly by the child's paediatrician, an ENT specialist, an eye specialist and a surgeon, but once at school the child comes under the care of school physicians who are all members of the staff of the local children's polyclinic.

SUPERVISION OF SCHOOL HEALTH SERVICE AND OTHER
CHILDREN'S ESTABLISHMENTS

A national network of crèches, nurseries and kindergartens has been built up in the USSR to enable mothers of young children to return to work, and it has been estimated that the following proportion of children attend these establishments (parents pay small fees to send children to these pre-school establishments):

Children aged 0–0·9 year – 10 per cent attend crèches
Children aged 1–2·9 years – 25 per cent attend nurseries
Children aged.3–6·9 years – 75 per cent attend kindergartens
Children aged 7 years   – all commence school.

However, these rates vary very much in different areas, and a report in *The Times* of London on 8 March 1968 noted that, in 1967, only 23 per cent of pre-school children in Moscow could attend nurseries or kindergartens on account of a shortage of both premises and staff.

With all these organised facilities the care and health of Soviet children has improved greatly over the past fifty years but qualitatively it still has room for improvement. For example there is still a high incidence of rheumatic fever, quoted in 1967 to be 10 per 1,000 children (under age of 15) a rate some ten times those prevalent in the USA and the UK.

Maternity and Child Care in the USA

Again, in America the pattern of maternity and child health and welfare services depends very largely on social, economic and geographical factors.

MATERNITY

Almost all deliveries are carried out in hospitals under the direction and supervision of a physician, and it is not customary for a midwife to take charge of a delivery, except in poor areas where there is an acute shortage of physicians.

Patients may have private care by a recognised specialist obstetrician with a board certificate, or from a 'specialoid' obstetrician who also works as a doctor-of-first-contact for other conditions. They may be looked after through a pre-paid insurance shceme by a medical group, of whom one or more members may be obstetricians (it should be noted that most hospital pre-paid insurance schemes exclude payment for obstetrics), or else State or local public hospitals for poor medical indigents. General care during the pre-natal and postnatal period is provided also for the poor through the local public health services.

The form of antenatal care is of the traditional pattern with regular monthly, or more frequent, examinations and with instruction on hygiene and mothercraft. Although all planned deliveries are conducted in hospitals or maternity homes in the USA, the period of stay in hospital is very short in uncomplicated and normal cases, 1–3 days, to reduce costs.

There is a high rate of operative interference in US obstetric practice. Almost all women have an episiotomy (cutting of the perineal tissues); many have a 'low forceps extraction' and many are given anaesthesia either by inhalation, through the spinal column (epidural or spinal) or by extensive skin infiltration with a local anaesthetic. Caesarean section is also frequent (around 10 per cent of deliveries). All such procedures are carried out by the obstetrician who is present and delivers almost all normal, as well as abnormal, cases.

The reasons for the high rate of operative interference and the presence of the physician at delivery may be traditional, but it is likely that another explanation is the fee-for-service system of private care, where the patient pays the physician for services rendered and expects him to be there to conduct the delivery.

Postnatal stay in hospital is short and is, as noted, often no longer than 1–3 days, even in the case of Caesarean section, but at home there are no special arrangements for postnatal supervision and the obstetrician does not visit routinely, although available if there are any complications.

QUALITATIVE INDICES OF MATERNITY CARE

Some of the qualitative indices of maternity care in the AUS are shown in Table 33.

TABLE 33

Qualitative indices of maternity care in the USA

Birth rate per 1,000	Maternal mortality per 100,000 births	Infant mortality per 1,000 births	Illegitimacy rate per 100 births
19·4	31	25	6·9

(Source: US Bureau of the Census, *U.S.A. 1967.*)

In general legalised abortion is not available in the USA but it is possible to carry out a termination of pregnancy for the ill-health of the mother, provided the circumstances are serious enough.

CHILD CARE

The patterns of child care in the USA depend on the mother's circumstances and, like antenatal care, may be private care, by a specialist paediatrician; by a specialoid first-contact paediatrician; by a general practitioner; or public care from the local public health and hospital services.

It comprises care for the sick child at the hospital, clinic or office – home visits are discouraged and are unusual; regular supervision of the healthy child at clinic or office; and preventive inoculations. There is no rigid or set routine, each physician and unit arranging their own programme.

Similarly, care for the school child is also a mixture of

services, depending on the school and its situation. In some areas the school health service carries out regular examinations of all children and supervision of their progress, but in others such services have lapsed because of staff shortages.

The health of the American child tends to be fairly good, although there are marked differences amongst the social groups.

If we consider again the frequency of rheumatic fever, for example, it is found that the annual incidence for children (under 15) was 1·5 per 1,000 in 1967.

Maternity and Child Care in the UK

All persons in the UK are entitled to register with and receive care from a general medical practitioner, and it is the woman's general practitioner who makes the initial diagnosis of pregnancy, confirmed if necessary by a pregnancy test carried out for him at the local hospital's laboratory. Having established that his patient is pregnant, the general practitioner then discusses the possible arrangements for maternity care with the mother.

At present more than three out of every four births in the UK take place in a hospital and this proportion is increasing each year. Nevertheless one-quarter of births take place in the woman's own home, either because of preference or because of local shortages of maternity beds. Those who are delivered at home are women who have had previous normal pregnancies and those whose home conditions are suitable. Priorities for hospital confinement include first pregnancy, any abnormality of present or past pregnancy, fourth pregnancy onwards, rhesus negative blood group of mother, poor social conditions and strong preference by the mother.

The general practitioner may be wholly responsible for the expectant mother who is to be delivered at home or at a general practitioner maternity hospital unit. In providing such supervision, for which he is paid extra fees, the GP works closely with the district midwife who also supervises the expectant mother and who carries out the actual normal delivery, the physician being called in if any abnormality occurs.

Maternity and Child Care

The general practitioner may also carry out antenatal care for women booked for hospital confinement, when the patient attends the GP's clinic until the thirty-sixth week and then returns to the care of the hospital's clinic (the GP receives extra fees for such services). Not all general practitioners provide such services and it is left entirely to the GP to decide.

The Local Authority through its public health department is involved with domiciliary obstetrics. It employs district midwives, who supervise the antenatal care of all mothers booked for home confinements, carry out normal home deliveries and undertake postnatal care for fourteen days. They now also care postnatally for women who are discharged early (after 2–3 days) from hospital. The district midwives work from their own clinics which usually are separate from GP premises. At these clinics in addition to antenatal care mothers are given mothercraft education and instruction in relaxation and psychoprophylaxis.

The local authority, through the midwife, also supplies free many of the facilities and equipment required for home confinements.

The maternity units and hospitals are administratively separate from the other two services. The maternity departments are directed by specialist obstetricians, and antenatal care in hospitals is carried out by midwives and physicians. The mothers are seen monthly either at hospital or by their general practitioner, and then weekly from the thirty-second week.

Delivery of normal cases in hospital is conducted by midwives, the obstetricians and the junior medical staff are called in only to deal with abnormal situations. Analgesia is by inhalational means or use of drugs. The forceps rate is around 5–10 per cent in hospital practice and less than 1 per cent in domiciliary practice. The Caesarean section rate is now around 5 per cent of all hospital deliveries. The average post-natal stay in UK maternity hospital units is 7–8 days, but 20 per cent are now hospitalised for less than 3 days. Postnatal examination is carried out by the obstetrician or general practitioner 6 weeks after delivery.

The special features of maternity care in the UK are undoubtedly the important place of the midwife in carrying out the great majority of normal obstetrics; the existence of obstetric flying squads based on hospitals, which go out to resuscitate obstetric emergencies in the home; and the regular publication of Confidential Reports of Maternal Mortality by the Department of Health, which are critical analyses of such deaths and which consider how they might have been prevented.

Social legislation exists whereby expectant mothers receive grants during their pregnancies, the amounts depend on whether they were working until they became pregnant and whether the confinement takes place at home; in such cases extra monies are given. There are also special social services and assistance for unmarried mothers.

TABLE 34

Qualitative indices of maternity care in the UK

Birth rate per 1,000 births	Maternal mortality per 100,000	Infant mortality per 1,000 births	Illegitimacy rate per 100 births
18·4	25	20	7·2

(Sources: Reports of Ministry of Health for 1966 for England and Wales.)

CHILD CARE

Care of children in the UK is shared also by the three parts of the NHS with considerable overlapping and duplication of services. Many general practitioners now provide and organise special services and clinics for children under their care. The general practitioner with 2,500 persons on his list may have up to 500–700 children under the age of 15. In providing this child care and welfare, including well-baby care, immunisations, health education and care for sick children, some general practitioners now have the assistance of health visitors and nurses who are attached to their practices.

Local Authority Children's Clinics exist for similar purposes, except that sick children are not treated but referred to their own general practitioners. This duplication is necessary at present because not all general practitioners provide special care for their child patients and they are not encouraged or directed to do so. In these circumstances services have to be provided to ensure that *all* children receive care. Special services are provided also by local authorities for schools where children are examined periodically by school physicians and for mentally and physically handicapped children.

Hospital services for children are designed primarily to deal with the more major diseases. They are staffed by specialist paediatricians who combine care for in-patients with that for out-patient ambulatory cases who are referred to them by general practitioners.

Some Comparison of the Nations' Care

MATERNITY CARE

The basic elements of good maternity care are accepted in the three nations. These are regular antenatal care and supervision; delivery by specialists (obstetrician or midwife), preferably in hospital or special unit; and postnatal care and examination smoothly leading into the child welfare programme. Added to this medical scheme are special social aids and welfare benefits for the expectant mother, the nature and size of which vary in the three nations.

In the USSR there is a well-planned service for maternity care based on the Women's Consultation Centre and maternity hospitals in larger cities, and on polyclinics and district hospitals in smaller towns and on the feldsher–midwife and local hospital in rural areas. The maternity service is distinct from other hospital and polyclinic departments and within it there is separation, in the large cities, of in-patient and out-patient care. The care is free to all mothers and is provided by obstetricians and midwives. Delivery is almost always at hospital. The forceps or vacuum extractor rate is 3–4 per cent of all deliveries and that for Caesarean section 2–3 per cent of all deliveries (quoted in Leningrad in 1967 to WHO seminar). Postnatally there is a smooth transition to paediatric care provided at the polyclinics.

In the USA there is a multiplicity of systems of maternity care. There are few skilled midwives and almost all deliveries, certainly in private practice, are carried out by the physician.

The forceps and extractor rates are high, up to 50–75 per cent in some units and so are the rates for Caesarean section, around 10 per cent of all deliveries.

In the UK under a National Health Service which has carried on many past traditions, maternity care is still shared between the three parts of the service, i.e. general practice, public health and hospital. One quarter of all deliveries still take place in the patients' homes and midwives are responsible for most normal deliveries. The current rates for operative interference are 10 per cent for forceps or vacuum extraction and 5 per cent for Caesarean section.

AN EVALUATION

There are many similarities and a few differences in the three nations (Tables 35 and 36).

The indices of birth rate, maternal and infant mortalities are similar in all three, as are illegitimacy rates in the USA and the UK. Although some deliveries still take place at home in the UK the trend is progressively towards hospital care. The lengths of stay are longer in the USSR and the UK than in the USA and the rates of operative interference rise from the lowest of Russia's to the highest in America. Divorce rates, similar in the USSR and the USA are higher than in the UK.

TABLE 35

Some indices of maternity care

	Birth rate per 1,000	Maternal mortality per 100,000 births	Infant mortality per 1,000 births	Illegitimacy per 100 births	Divorce per 1,000	per 100 marriages
USSR	18·4	32	28	One legalised abortion per birth (No other data available.)	2	18
USA	19·4	31	25	6·9	2·5	25
UK	18·4	25	20	7·2	0·7	11

TABLE 36

Hospitalisation and operative interference data in maternity care

| | Deliveries in hospital per 100 births | Average stay in hospital (days) | Operative interference per 100 births | |
			Forceps and vacuum extraction	Caesarean section
USSR	100	8–9	3–4	2–3
USA	100	3–4	Up to 50–75 in some units	10
UK	75	7–8	10	5

Apart from these there are no qualitative differences in maternity care as judged by the maternal and infant mortality rates.

CHILD CARE

Modern child care comprises services for the well-child, preventive measures and the sick child.

In Soviet Russia integration of these measures has been achieved through the co-operation of polyclinics and hospital units, but in America the care is shared between private specialist and 'specialoid' care and that provided by local public health services and hospitals for the less affluent.

In the U.K. care of the sick child is shared between the general practitioner and the hospital, and preventive and supervisory care for healthy children is shared between the general practitioner and the public health services.

As far as can be ascertained it seems that it is not the pattern of organisation of services that plays the major part in the health of children, but rather the level of national social development and advancement.

The USSR has a plentiful supply of physicians, nurses, polyclinics and hospitals but the incidence of socio-medical diseases such as rheumatic fever, tuberculosis and infections of the digestive tract in children is still higher than it is in either America or the United Kindgom.

Chapter 10
Mental Health Care

Mental illness is one of the 'new' conditions that have filled the vacuum created by the control of 'old' diseases. Whether the increase has been real or apparent is uncertain but the facts are that modern medical care at all levels has to be prepared and able to manage more of these disorders than in the past. The increase has occurred in the psychoneuroses as distinct from the more severe psychoses, and within the psychoneuroses it is the affective disorders, and in particular depression, that has increased in step with social advance and better standards of health and welfare.

Techniques of care for the mentally ill have changed dramatically over the past twenty years. Altered attitudes of both public and profession have been one advance, but in addition great progress has been made in psychopharmacology and many new and effective drugs have become available for all grades and types of mental illness.

Community care measures designed to help in the rehabilitation of the patient and in support for the family are becoming more necessary with the expansion of services and create problems of themselves in staffing and effective utilisation.

It is in the midst of these changing situations that the mental health services of the USSR, the USA and the UK have to be considered.

The Care of the Mentally Ill in the USSR

The Soviet attitude to mental illness is that it presents fewer problems in a 'socialist' culture than in so-called 'capitalist' societies. It is stated that because of Soviet social achievements the prevalence of mental illness is low and will decrease further because of further social and cultural improvements.

Such a national attitude influences profoundly the pattern of medical services created to deal with the mentally sick. In the face of such attitudes it becomes almost a slur to suffer from a mental illness, because it will let down the image of a happy society. For this reason it is difficult to obtain facts and data on the true prevalence of mental illness in the USSR. The data that is available, however, suggests that the prevalence of mental illness in the USSR is very much of the same order as in the USA and the UK (*vide infra*). The therapeutic approach to mental illness is influenced by these national and cultural attitudes. Psycho-analysis is frowned upon and psychopharmacology has been slow to develop but great emphasis has been placed on Pavlovian principles of conditioning particularly in association with group therapy.

Field (1967) refers to a study of morbidity carried out in the USSR and quotes the rates for mental and nervous illnesses shown in Table 37.

TABLE 37

Annual prevalence of morbidity of psychoses and nervous diseases per 1,000 in the USSR

Disease	Male	Female	All
Psychoses	5·7	3·1	4·2
Diseases of the nervous sytem	57·9	59·7	58·9
All diseases	1,198·2	1,036·7	1,106·1

(Source: Field, M.G., in *New Aspects of Mental Health Services*, Pergamon Press, London (1967).)

The prevalence rate of 63·1 per 1,000 of all 'nervous' and psychiatric illnesses in the USSR is thus not dissimilar from that of the USA and the UK, but the almost equal distribution in the two sexes is very different. In the USA and the UK the prevalence of mental illness is much higher in females than in males.

THE PATTERN OF CARE

Care for the common and less serious mental illnesses is provided by the local physicians at the polyclinics, and the conditions treated here are the many personal and personality problems that can be managed so well by a physician who knows his patients from long-term experience. If the *uchastok* physician requires more expert assistance the patient is referred either to a 'neuropathologist' (psychiatrist) at the polyclinic, who is able to undertake short-term or long-term care, or, in a large city, to a 'psychiatric dispensary'. This is a special polyclinic that deals only with the mentally sick, and is staffed by psychiatrists, some of whom are also on the staff of the local mental hospital.

Patients have direct access to these dispensaries and can by-pass the local physicians and attend the psychiatric dispensary of their own volition. There are facilities at such dispensaries for the long-term support of ambulatory patients and arrangements can be made to admit patients for treatment in mental hospitals. Psychiatrists and nurses at the psychiatric dispensaries may visit patients in their homes and there are also facilities for day-care, some beds being available at the dispensary for short-term care and assessment. It is the role of these dispensaries to provide a community psychiatric service for up to 400,000 of the population who reside in the area. Within each dispensary region there are *uchastoks* (neighbourhood areas) of some 40,000, each in turn under the care of a district psychiatrist.

These district psychiatrists are expected to come to know the people in their area who need or may come to need psychiatric and psychosocial aid, and each psychiatrist works with one nurse who acts as a social worker and assistant.

THE MENTAL HOSPITAL

The structure and design of Soviet mental hospitals is similar to those of the USA and the UK and they tend to be large and situated often some distance away from the city centres. Within the hospital standard care with anti-depressant and psychotropic drugs is available and in addition physical methods including electroconvulsive therapy, hydrotherapy and physiotherapy are used.

The patients in the Soviet mental hospital are grouped and warded according to certain common characteristics such as their age, sex and stage and nature of disease, and there are special wards for the physically sick, medico-legal, military, convalescent and other groups of cases. Most of the wards in Soviet mental hospitals are still 'closed' and locked but there are moves to relax these restrictions. In common with trends elsewhere there has been reported a fall in the average length of stay per person in hospital in the past decade from 180–200 days to 60–70 days.

Table 38 shows the psychiatric facilities available in the USSR.

TABLE 38

Psychiatric facilities in the USSR

PHYCHIATRISTS

Percentage of all physicians	Population per psychiatrist	Psychiatrists per 100,000
4·5%	11,100	9

PSYCHIATRIC HOSPITAL BEDS

Per 1,000 of population	Percentage of all hospital beds	Ratio of psychiatric to non-psychiatric beds	Persons per bed
0·93*	11·5%	1 : 7·7	1,002

Public psychiatric beds per psychiatrist	Psychiatric staff : patients	Psychiatrist per patients in hospital
27·7	1 : 1	1 : 27

* Planned to rise to 2·0.

(Sources: Craft, M., and Field, M.G., in *New Aspects of Mental Health Services*, Pergamon Press, London (1967).)

The Care of the Mentally Ill in the USA

It is readily recognised and accepted that in the USA the problem of mental illness is creating an increasing challenge to modern medical care, and steps are slowly being taken to meet it. In the past this challenge has not been fully accepted, and whilst provisions were made to cope with the major psychoses that required long-term institutional care, no arrangements were organised to provide a system of care for less severe grades of mental illness. Even less was provided for mental illness than for non-psychiatric illnesses. Psychi-

atric care (along with maternity care) has been specifically
excluded from many prepaid insurance shemes and no
special arrangements have been made to organise area
services to cover needs for mental care.

Other difficulties exist because of the traditional free-
enterprise system of American life. Of 15,000 psychiatrists in
the USA two-thirds are involved with private practice, and
one-fifth of these work exclusively in private practice and
are not available for non-private work. (Joint Information
Service of American Psychiatric Association and National
Association for Mental Health, Fact Sheet No. 10, 1959.)
Less than one-third of these psychiatrists (4,350) work either
part time or full time in the State and Federal Service to
help in the care of the more severe forms of mental illness.
The majority are involved in private care of the less major
psychiatric disorders.

The true extent of mental illness in the USA is unknown
but expressed as physician consultation rates, the annual
prevalence rates, for all mental illness, are between 35 and
40 per 1,000 (Densen, P., *et al.* (1960), *Milbank Mem. Fund
Quart.*, *38*, 48 and Huntley, R. (1963), *J. Amer. Med.
Assoc.*). These reports were based on the work of doctors-of-
first-contact and represent the rates for those who were able
to, and felt it necessary to attend their primary physicians
for advice and help. According to Field (1967) the prevalence
rate for 'psychoses' in the USA is between 5 and 7 per 1,000.

THE PATTERN OF CARE

There is no single simple system of care for mental illness
in the USA and a great variety of possibilities exist depending
on the locale, the facilities available and the socio-economic
standing of the patient. It is at the first level of contact that
care for the majority of mental illness, which is of the less
serious type, is provided by the various doctors-of-first-
contact. These primary physicians are, as has been noted
in Chapter 4, of various types and they also are inevitably
involved in the care of such patients, intentionally or uninten-
tionally, and willingly or unwillingly, for the simple reason
that these conditions account for so much of the work of
all branches of medical care.

There is a conspicuous lack of resources at the level

of specialist ambulatory care. There are a few organised schemes for specialist psychiatric care, but in most areas there are no such facilities. There is a relative shortage of psychiatrists; they are not uniformly distributed over the USA, most are segregated along the densely populated Eastern and Western seaboards; and most schemes of mental care that do exist are for private patients.

MENTAL HOSPITALS

Most American mental hospitals are large and situated far away from city centres. They are still associated with, and geared for the old and traditional custodial roles for long-term care. Such roles are changing however, and the hospitals are becoming more concerned with the shorter-stay case (the average length of stay has fallen from 83 days in 1950 to 50 days in 1964) no doubt as a direct result of new and more successful forms of therapy.

Most of the American mental hospitals are administered by Federal and State Authorities, but there are also some small private mental hospitals and clinics often owned and administered by psychiatrists themselves.

A more recent trend has been for the larger general hospitals, particularly university hospitals, to establish psychiatric units and wards within the general framework to try and avoid the segregation of the mentally sick in the old-type mental hospitals.

The fragmentation of care in the USA into private and non-private sectors has made any attempts to establish overall community care for the mentally ill extremely difficult.

The psychiatric facilities available in the USA are shown in Table 39.

TABLE 39

Facilities for mental illness – psychiatrists and psychiatric hospital beds in the USA

PSYCHIATRISTS

Percentage of all physicians	Population per psychiatrist	Psychiatrists per 100,000
5%	13,500	7–8

TABLE 39—*cont.*

PSYCHIATRIC HOSPITAL BEDS

Per 1,000	Percentage of all hospital beds	Psychiatric to non-psychiatric	Persons per bed	Public psychiatric beds per psychiatrist
4·0	46·4%	1 : 1·16	238	183·9

Psychiatric staff : patients	Patients in psychiatric hospital per psychiatrist
1 : 4	184 : 1

(Sources: Craft (1967) and Field (1967).)

The Care of the Mentally Ill in the UK

The challenges of mental illness are being met in the UK through a variety of measures. Public attitudes have changed very much in the past twenty years and the Mental Health Act of 1959 has created a more liberal approach to legislation associated with mental illness. The public tolerance to mental illness has changed and the mentally sick in both acute and chronic states are much more acceptable within the community. Sufferers are more ready and prepared to seek advice for mental illnesses that have become more 'respectable' than in the past and there is less fear of hospitalisation. The image of mental hospitals has altered. No longer is there fear of being admitted and 'locked up'. Few mental wards are now closed (locked). The NHS has created opportunities for placing the care of the mentally sick on a community basis and these opportunities have led to a better service.

A number of investigations have been carried out in the UK to assess the prevalence and nature of mental illness in the community (summarised by Shepherd, M., Cooper, B., Brown, H.C., and Kalton, G.W., in *Psychiatric Illness in General Practice*, Oxford University Press, London (1966)). From these studies it is suggested that the total prevalence of mental illness at the first-contact levels is between 50 and 150 per 1,000, varying with area, the physician and criteria used. The prevalence of psychoses is around 5–6 per 1,000.

189

Looked at in another way, it is evident that between 10 and 15 per cent of the work of the first-contact general practitioner is concerned with the management of definite mental illnesses.

THE PATTERN OF CARE

The three parts of the NHS are involved in the care of the mentally sick, but the greatest amount of work falls on the general practitioner and the psychiatrist. He manages a great deal of mental illness himself, in a general supportive fashion and without the use of special techniques or training and refers to the specialist psychiatrist only a small minority (5 per cent) of diagnosed cases (Shepherd *et al.* (1966)).

There is an increasing degree of involvement by the community services of the local authorities, whereby mental welfare officers, hostels and day centres are provided and there is more evidence of closer co-operation with hospital and general practitioner services. The specialist ambulatory services are organised by the local hospital authorities and are staffed by psychiatrists working at psychiatric hospitals, or from the out-patient department of general hospitals.

The facilities available for the care of mental illnesses in the UK are shown in Table 40.

TABLE 40

Facilities for mental health care in the UK

PSYCHIATRISTS

Percentage of all physicians	Population per psychiatrist*	Psychiatrist* per 100,000
5%	18,000	5–6

PSYCHIATRIC HOSPITAL BEDS

Per 1,000	Percentage of all Hospital beds	Psychiatric to non-psychiatric beds	Persons per psychiatric bed
4·0	44%	1 : 1·3	240

TABLE 40—*cont.*

Psychiatric beds per psychiatrist	Staff : patient	Patients per psychiatrist (specialist)
93	1 :3·5	1 :175

* *Psychiatrist* include all grades of physicians working as psychiatrists, including junior hospital staff.

(Source: Report of Ministry of Health for 1966.)

Comparisons of Care

The current prevalence rates of mental disease are not very different in the three countries. (Table 41.)

TABLE 41

Prevalence of mental diseases in rates per 1,000 from USSR, USA and UK sources

	USSR	USA	UK
Psychoses	4	6	6
'Psychoneurosis'	59	53	89
TOTAL	63	59	95

Excluding 'psychosomatic' ailments which in the USA and the UK have prevalence rates of 40 per 1,000.

(Sources: Shepherd *et al.* (1966) and Field (1967).)

These rates must be taken as guides only because comparison depends very much on the criteria and definitions used and these are certainly not uniform. What the rates do confirm is that mental illnesses are a major source of common morbidity that requires special services to meet the needs of care.

Differences in approach are notable. In the USSR it is intended to double the proportion of hospital beds for mental illness, whereas in the USA and the UK the plans are to reduce the numbers of such beds. The explanation is probably that in the USA and the UK there was an over-supply for long stay cases in the past fifty years and now, with new forms of therapy such long stays are no longer required. In the USSR beds for mental illness did not have priority in the early days of the pre- and post-revolutionary periods and only now is the system developing to meet the needs with more realism.

PATTERNS OF CARE

The modern aim of mental care is to keep the patient within his own family and home environment wherever possible, and to restrict hospitalisation to short periods for specific forms of therapy. However, it is realised that some long-term chronic and incurable cases will occur and will require permanent custodial care, and facilities have to be provided for them.

In the USSR and the UK increasing co-operation between first-contact ambulatory specialist and hospital services has led to the evolution of a certain basic pattern of care. Modern management of mental diseases requires the establishment of local community services based on populations of from 50,000 to 500,000 persons, depending on the density of the population. This pattern that has evolved comprises care by the first-contact health team of general physicians and paramedical auxiliaries, and the majority of mental illnesses are cared for in fact at this level. According to Shepherd *et al.* (1966) only 5 per cent of such cases in the UK are referred by the GP to a specialist. Specialist services exist to care for the more difficult psychoneuroses and for most

TABLE 42

Comparisons of facilities for mental illnesses in the USSR, the USA and the UK

	USSR	USA	UK
Psychiatrists per 100,000	9	7–8	5–6
Psychiatric hospital beds per 1,000	0·93	4·0	4·0
Psychiatric hospital beds per psychiatrist	27	187	175

psychoses. Such services work from their own units which combine out-patient and in-patient departments. Specialist psychiatrists are supported by psychiatric social and welfare workers and nurses.

Such progression as has occurred in the USSR and the UK is not apparent in the USA, not because the idea of community care is unacceptable, but because of the inherent system of free-enterprise medical care.

Table 42 shows that proportionately the USSR has more psychiatrists and fewer psychiatric hospital beds than the USA and the UK, and in consequence Soviet psychiatrists have many fewer patients in hospital to care for.

A Personal Evaluation

It is becoming clear that corresponding with the development of modern social and medical advances and an easier, more comfortable and longer life, the prevalence of mental illness is nevertheless increasing and creating problems of management and care. It is not possible to think in terms of 'cure' in mental illness. The cause of many mental illnesses depends on unalterable personality and environmental characteristics and although it may be possible, with treatment, to make the two factors more compatible with fewer symptoms, personal suffering and family distress, permanent 'cure' is unlikely. Services have to be planned, therefore, to provide long-term care of vulnerable individuals and families, and social as well as medical measures, must be included in any system trying to prevent recurrences and breakdown.

To meet such a difficult and challenging situation all levels of medical care must be brought into a co-operatively organised community service. In such a service the doctor-of-first-contact will have an important role in providing support and care for the less serious disorders that account for most mental illness – but the specialist services must be available to be brought in when necessary, not only in the care of established cases but in planning preventive and educational approaches for the community.

Chapter 11
The Greater Medical Profession

The use that is made of a country's medical manpower is of supreme importance. Changing patterns of care including closer collaboration and better team work, have led to some rethinking of the roles and functions of various members of the 'greater medical profession'. In addition to physicians there are the middle-grade paramedical auxiliaries, including nurses, medical technologists and social workers. They, with the primary physician, form the health team, and their training, attitudes and responsibilities profoundly influence the quality of care that can be achieved by a nation's medical manpower.

The Medical Manpower of the USSR

PHYSICIANS

At the end of 1965 there were 550,000 physicians in active practice in Soviet Russia (Table 43), and of these 70 per cent per women.

TABLE 43

Physicians in the USSR

Population	230 million
Number of physicians	480,000* (excluding 70,000 dental surgeons)
Physicians per population	1 : 480
Physicians per 10,000	21 per 10,000

* 70 per cent women.

The Greater Medical Profession

A breakdown of physicians according to their specialities (Table 44) shows that one-quarter of them act as first-contact doctors, i.e. as local therapists and paediatricians, 60 per cent are in recognised clinical specialities and that the remaining 15 per cent comprise public health physicians (hygienists) (8 per cent), administrators and other non-clinical categories.

TABLE 44

Proportions of Physicians in various specialities in the USSR in 1965

	%
Doctors-of-first-contact (local physicians)	25
Medical specialities (including general medicine, paediatrics, tuberculosis and infectious diseases, radiology and pathology)	30
Surgical specialities (including general surgery, ENT, ophthalmology orthopaedics and anaesthetics)	25
Psychiatrists and neurologists	5
Others (including public health and administration)	15
TOTAL	100

Dental surgeons and dental assistants are generally included as 'physicians' but this is not customary in the USA and the UK. In the USSR, in 1965, there were 26,000 dental surgeons (1.1 per 10,000 population) and 44,000 dental assistants (1.9 per 10,000).

Between 1950 and 1965 the total numbers of physicians doubled from 237,000 to 480,000 respectively (Ryan, T.M. (1968), *Medical Practitioners Union News Letter*, *19*, 6–6, quoting Narodnoe Khozyaistvo v. 1965 of Moscow 1966). The proportionate increases varied with specialities. The greatest increases were for psychiatrists, with a rise of 250 per cent and for radiologists a 237 per cent increase. Tuberculosis specialists more than doubled (130 per cent) but specialists in dermatology and venereology remained almost the same (increase of 12 per cent) in number, and physicians in the public health service increased by 66 per cent (compared with overall increase of 107 per cent for all physicians).

Geographical Distribution

The difficulties in staffing rural, outlying and less socially desirable areas with physicians are evident from the variations of rates of physicians per 10,000 of the population.

Whereas European Soviet Republics such as Georgia (34·6 physicians per 10,000), Latvia (31·4), Estonia (29·8), Armenia (27·2), Russia (24·9) and Ukraine (24·3), have rates above that for the whole Union 23·9 (including dental surgeons and assistants), those for the outlying Asiatic Republics as Tadzhik (14·9), Uzbek (16·9), Kayakh (18·4) and Kirgiz (18·8) are considerably lower. (Ryan, T.M., 1968.) Other data show that whilst only 7 per cent of urban appointments for physicians are unfilled, 16 per cent of those in rural areas remain unfilled. This state exists in spite of the fact that 40 per cent of all new medical graduates are directed into rural areas for the first three years of their postgraduate periods.

MIDDLE GRADE MEDICAL WORKERS

At the end of 1965 there were 1·8 million 'middle-grade medical workers' in the USSR or 78·5 per 10,000 of the population. These middle-grade workers were trained personnel serving as assistants to physicians.

The various groupings are shown in Table 45.

The nursing staff situation in the USSR corresponds closely to that of other nations, where most (three out of four) work in hospitals, the remainder in peripheral units, such as polyclinics or dispensaries. The status of the nurse in the USSR is rather lowly compared with feldshers and because of the relatively large numbers of physicians they do not undertake many of the duties undertaken by trained nurses in the USA and the UK.

Feldshers are a special category of middle-grade medical personnel, unique to the USSR. This grade is a multi-purpose one and feldshers work in many medical and social spheres in close collaboration with and responsible to a physi-

TABLE 45

Middle-grade medical workers in the USSR

Types	Rates per 10,000
Nurses (all types)	33·9 (3 out of 4 nurses work in hospitals)
Feldshers	17·1
Feldsher–midwives	3·4
Midwives	7·4
Radiographers (X-ray assistants)	0·9
Laboratory assistants	2·8
Sanitary assistants	1·3
Disinfectors	2·9
Dental technicians	0·8

Pharmacists
  Fully trained   1·6 ⎫
  Partly trained   3·9 ⎭
	5·5

Others	2·5
TOTAL	78·5 (1·83 million)

cian. Historically the feldsher was a military invention of the seventeenth century. Peter the Great was faced with a shortage of trained physicians for his campaigns and he therefore introduced lay medical assistants, quickly trained by physicians, who acted as military field surgeons. In the nineteenth century, following the abolition of serfdom, the concept of the feldsher was introduced into civil life and the first feldshers were those who had served as such in the armies. Because of the shortage of physicians, feldshers had to undertake many duties for which they were untrained, but there was no one else to do this work. The feldsher, in poorer and rural areas especially, became a second-rate 'physician'. With the Revolution in 1917 abolition of the feldsher grade was considered, but it was realised that they filled an essential role, provided that they did not undertake duties for which they were not trained and provided that they worked in association with, and under the direction of, a physician. There are now 400,000 feldshers and 80,000 feldsher–midwives in the USSR, and there are 75,000 feldsher posts in rural areas – but only one-half of feldshers work in rural areas. The feldsher in the USSR today is a specially trained multi-purpose middle-grade medical worker, not a second-rate physician. Her work is defined specifically and is organised so that she works in association with and under the direction of physicians. In rural areas feldshers and feldsher–midwives are based in collective farms and villages, and under medical supervision their work includes care of minor medical problems, supervision and follow-up of more major disorders under the direction of the physician, preventive care, including immunisation and pre-symptomatic screening, health education and general sanitary and hygienic duties. In the cities, feldshers are more specialised and may be attached to polyclinics, industrial units, ambulances, public health departments (sanepids), laboratories or to special dispensaries dealing with tuberculosis, mental illnesses, cancer or other diseases.

THE HEALTH TEAM

In the hospitals physicians and nurses work together in traditional ways but there is less delegation of tasks to nurses. The nurse in the USSR primarily nurses the sick, and physicians carry out technical diagnostic and therapeutic procedures. Feldshers have few roles in hospital work.

In the community some attempts are being made to group local physicians into larger units in urban polyclinics but there is no evidence of any real incorporation of feldshers into such groups. Bedevilling the development of family health teams is the separation of the services for children, adults and specific diseases. Until general polyclinics are established where care for the whole family can be provided by a single group of medical personnel, then the evolution of realistic and useful health teams will be difficult. Each polyclinic physician has a personal nurse working with him, and she combines the role of receptionist, clerk and secretary as well as nurse but as in the hospital service carries out few technical procedures.

Medical Manpower in the USA

PHYSICIANS

At the end of 1965 there were 297,000 physicians in the USA. Of these 286,000 were doctors of medicine and 11,000 doctors of osteopathy recognised as qualified to practise medicine. (Table 46.)

TABLE 46
Physicians in the USA

Population	200 million
Number of physicians	297,000
Physicians per population	1 : 670
Physicians per 10,000	15 per 10,000

The proportionate increase in numbers since 1950 was from 221,000 in 1950 to 297,000 in 1965, an increase of one-third (34 per cent). Of all physicians in active practice in 1965 the breakdown in specialities is shown in Table 4 according to *Health Manpower Perspective 1967* (USA Public Health Service Publication No. 1667, Washington, 1967).

TABLE 47
Proportions of US physicians in various specialities

	%
Doctors-of-first-contact (including general practitioners and specialoids)	40
Medical specialities	20
Surgical specialities	30
Psychiatrists and neurologists	5
Others	5
TOTAL	100

(Source: *Health Manpower Perspective*, 1967.)

The proportion of first-contact physicians has fallen from 65 per cent in 1950 to 40 per cent in 1965 and the proportions in full specialities have risen accordingly. In 1965 there were in the USA 95,400 dental surgeons (4·7 per 10,000), 16,000 dental hygienists (0·8 per 10,000) and 95,000 dental assistants (4·7 per 10,000).

Geographical Distribution

There is a great range in the distribution of physicians in the various States of America. Bearing in mind that the overall rate of physicians is 15 per 10,000, in Washington,

The Greater Medical Profession

DC, there are 36·7 physicians per 10,000, in the State of New York there are 21·1, in Connecticut 17·8 and in California 17·7. On the other hand there are many fewer in Alaska (6·6), Mississippi (7·4), South Dakota (7·8) and South Carolina (7·9). (Rates quoted in *U.S.A. 1967*, US Bureau of the Census 1967.)

MIDDLE-GRADE MEDICAL WORKERS

In 1965 there were 1·37 million middle-grade medical workers in the USA, a rate of 68·4 per 10,000. The proportions in the various categories are shown in Table 48.

TABLE 48

Middle-grade medical workers in the USA

	Rates per 10,000
Nurses	
Registered Nurses	32·0 (two-thirds work in hospitals and one-fifth in private practice)
Practical Nurses	15·0 (one-half work in hospitals)
Radiographers	3·6
Medical (laboratory) technicians	2·0
Dental technicians	1·3
Pharmacists	6·0
Others (including physiotherapists, occupational and speech therapists)	8·5
TOTAL	68·4

(Source: *Health Manpower Perspective*, 1967.)

In the categories of Table 48 'Nurses' are divided into 'registered' and 'practical', the difference being in their training programmes and qualifications. Registered nurses may be diplomates or degree holders with 2–5 years of training, whereas practical nurses need have only one year of recognised training. It will be noted that there are no midwives and no feldshers equivalents in the table.

The fee-for-service system does not encourage delegation and sharing of work between physician and paramedical workers. The physician therefore often undertakes tasks that may be carried out by others. This is particularly notable in the field of normal obstetrics where the almost total absence of recognised midwives involves physicians in much unnecessary work.

In the personal care of the patient, nurses in the USA undertake two distinct functions. They nurse the sick and they act as technicians and administrators. There is some ambivalence however towards personal nursing of the sick, and the more highly trained registered nurse, especially those with degree qualifications, appear rather reluctant to 'nurse' the sick, and is more interested in acting as nurse-technician and administrator. Personal nursing care, therefore, tends to be more in the hands of practical nurses who are less highly trained.

THE HEALTH TEAM

Apart from a few experimental ventures there has been little progress towards the concept of a 'health team', and the idea of a group of physicians working with and delegating responsibility to middle-grade medical colleagues has gained scant acceptance with physicians or with the public in the United States.

Medical Manpower in the UK

PHYSICIANS

At the end of 1965 there were 55,000 physicians in active practice in the UK. (Table 49.)

TABLE 49
Physicians in the UK

Population	50 million
Number of physicians	55,000
Physicians per population	1 : 900
Physicians per 10,000	11 per 10,000

(Source: *Medical Manpower*, Office of Health Economics, London (1966).)

Compared with 1950 the numbers of all active physicians has increased by one-third (33 per cent), and this increase has been much greater in the hospital field, where the number of specialists has doubled, whereas in general practice the increase has been less than one-sixth (15 per cent). The proportions in the various professional categories are as shown in Table 50.

TABLE 50

Proportions of UK physicians in various specialities

	%	
Doctors-of-first-contact (general practitioners)	40	
Medical specialities	20	
Surgical specialities	20	
Psychiatrists and neurologists	5	
Others	15	(public health, 5 per cent)
TOTAL	100	

Since 1950 the proportion of general practitioners has fallen from 45 per cent to 40 per cent of all active physicians, and the proportion in hospital specialities has risen from 30 per cent to 45 per cent.

In 1965 there were 10,500 dental surgeons (2·0 per 10,000) and the same number of dental hygienists and assistants (2·0 per 10,000).

Geographical Distribution

The United Kingdom is a small and densely populated island with a relatively even distribution of physicians but some variation does exist, for example, in general practice the range of general practitioners is from 3·7 per 10,000 or one for every 2,669 persons in the West Midlands, an industrial region, to 4·6 per 10,000 or one per 2,118 in the more rural South-west.

MIDDLE-GRADE MEDICAL WORKERS

In 1965 there were 357,000 middle-grade medical workers in the UK, a rate of 65 per 10,000. The proportions are shown in Table 51.

In the hospitals the State Registered Nurses are those who have undergone a three-year training period before being successful at examination. State Enrolled Nurses require

TABLE 51
Middle-grade medical workers in England and Wales

		Rates per 10,000
	HOSPITAL	
Nurses*		
State registered nurses (SRN)	27	(11 per 10,000 in training)
State enrolled nurses (SEN)	10	(3 per 10,000 in training)
Midwives	3	(1 per 10,000 in training)
Other		
middle-grade medical workers	6	(radiographers 1 per 10,000, laboratory technicians 2 per 10,000)
	COMMUNITY	
Home nurses	2	
District midwives	1·5	
Health visitors	1·5	
Other medical, social and welfare staff	3	
Pharmacists	5	
Others	6	
TOTAL	65	

* Excluding 12 per 10,000 'other nurses'.
(Source: Report of Ministry of Health for 1967.)

fewer school-leaving qualifications for acceptance and have a shorter period of training. Nursing in UK hospitals is now a combination of both grades on the staff, providing a mixture of personal nursing care and the completion of technical tasks of a diagnostic and therapeutic nature. Midwives under the supervision of obstetricians, undertake much of normal obstetrics, including antenatal care and delivery, and they participate in the conduct of abnormal cases with the obstetrician.

In the community there are four groups of middle-grade medical workers, almost all employed by local public health authorities. District (home) nurses visit patients in their homes and carry out routine nursing duties on housebound persons under the care of general practitioners, and a large proportion of their work is with old persons, chronic sick and handicapped, and the nursing of some acute illnesses such as cerebrovascular accidents, pneumonias, childhood fevers and surgical cases discharged from hospital. Although employed by the local authorities district nurses work under the direction of general practitioners and many are now attached to general practice units.

General practitioners are free to employ their own general practice nurses for work in their units. (There is a reimbursement scheme in existence.) The main work of these nurses is on the practice premises but some follow-up visits may be carried out to patients in their own homes.

Health Visitors in the UK are equivalent in many respects to public health nurses in the USA and feldshers in the USSR, and their main roles are in the maintenance of health, prevention af disease and health education. Originally concerned with children and expectant mothers, health visitors are now involved in the care of the whole population An increasing proportion (nearly 20 per cent) are now attached to general practices and work with the practice population under the direction of the general practitioners, although employed by the local authority. Their work in general practice is involved with antenatal care, child health and welfare, care of the aged, chronic sick and handicapped, with social and family problems and with any medical or mental disorders where the physician considers she may be of assistance as a medical social worker.

Domiciliary midwives share supervision of normal obstetrics in the home (25 per cent of deliveries in 1967 were at home), and are increasingly involved in postnatal care of early discharge (2–3 days) cases from maternity hospitals.

There are also various special social workers engaged in child welfare, care of old people, mentally sick, problem families and others who may be involved in joint care in the community with general practitioners and nurses.

THE HEALTH TEAM

In the United Kingdom co-operation and collaboration between physicians and the various paramedical workers is steadily increasing. Such collaboration has been traditional hospital practice for generations, but although it is new in general practice, it is spreading fast. With the attachment of health visitors, nurses and midwives to general practices, sharing of work is possible and new roles and functions are being developed.

It is in the community field that great strides have thus been made in the UK to develop the concept of the health team working together and sharing the care and responsibilities of individuals and families that are medically or socially sick.

This first-level health team is able to refer more complex problems to more specialised levels of care in hospital and community organisations, thus medical problems are referred to hospital out-patient departments (ambulant cases) for admission, whilst others may need referral to the special district departments which specialise in social problems of children, the aged, the mentally sick, the blind, the deaf and the physically handicapped, and others. It is from the first-level team that such cases are selectively referred for advice and help.

Some Comparisons of the Medical Manpower Situation in the Three Countries

If allowances are made for the difficulties in making comparisons from published data presented in different ways and without any clear definitions, then it is of interest to compare the medical and paramedical manpower rates quoted. Any such comparisons must be made with the due caution that what is a 'nurse' in the USSR may be an 'aide, orderly' in the USA and so excluded from middle medical grading, or 'other nursing staff' in the UK and likewise excluded.

Likewise with 'physicians', and until their work is analysed comparisons must be inevitably rather crude.

PHYSICIANS

The rates of 'active' physicians in the three nations are shown in Table 52. The 'activity' of the physicians is difficult to ascertain. Some may be working full-time in clinical work, some may be engaged part-time in research, academic and administrative duties, others may be retired but still on the medical register and yet others may be women doctors who select to work only a few hours each week. More definitive studies are required before true comparisons can be made and before the true manpower needs of developed societies can be estimated.

TABLE 52

Comparisons of rates of physicians and increases (1950–1965)
in the USSR, the USA and the UK

	USSR	USA	UK
Physicians per population	1 : 480	1 : 670	1 : 900
Physicians per 10,000	21	15	11
Percentage increases 1950–1965	103%	34%	33%

Table 52 shows that the USSR has twice as many physicians as the UK, with the USA almost exactly half-way between. Notably, whereas the total number of physicians increased by one-third in the USA and the UK, it doubled in the USSR between 1950 and 1965. Attempts to compare the proportion of physicians in the various specialist branches are made difficult once again because of lack of uniformity of definitions. This is particularly so with respect to the branch of first-contact care. Table 53 shows that more physicians were in this latter branch in the USA and the UK than in the USSR, which had more in medical and surgical specialities.

TABLE 53

Percentage proportions of physicians in various branches in the
USSR, USA and UK

	USSR	USA	UK
Doctors-of-first-contact	25	40	40
Medical specialities	30	20	20
Surgical specialities	25	30	20
Psychiatrists and neurologists	5	5	5
Others	15	5	15
TOTAL	100	100	100

DENTAL STAFF

There are many more qualified dental surgeons and supportive staff in the USA than in the USSR and the UK. (Table 54.)

TABLE 54

Dental manpower in the USSR, the USA and the UK
(rates per 10,000)

	USSR	USA	UK
Dental surgeons	1·1	4·7	2·0
Dental hygienists	—	0·8	} 2·0*
Dental assistants	1·9	4·7	
Dental technicians	0·8	1·3	1·0*
TOTAL	3·8	11·5	5·0

* Estimated.

Geographical Distribution

Comparing the quoted ranges of regional distribution of physicians in the USSR, the range between the highest and lowest regional rates of physicians in 1965 was three-fold in the USA this range was six-fold, whereas in the UK the difference was only one-third.

MIDDLE-GRADE MEDICAL WORKERS

Accepting the difficulties of definitive comparisons, Table 55 shows the rates per 10,000 in the three nations.

If 'nurses' and 'midwives' are taken together then the rates per 10,000 are similar, i.e. USSR 40·3, USA 45·0 and UK 49·5. The great differences between the three nations are in the 20·5 per 10,000 feldshers and feldsher–midwives in the USSR, which is far greater than the nearest equivalents of US public health nurses at 2·0 per 10,000 and UK health visitors and allied medical social workers at 5·5 per 10,000. Descriptions of the work of Soviet feldshers have been given and they are being fairly fully utilised, but one cannot help posing serious questions as to their real need in the manpower structure, particularly as the rate of physicians in the USSR is also high.

The difficulties referred to in attempting to make comparisons of manpower resources in the USSR, the USA and the UK make it apparent that there is much that is unknown of the exact work being carried out by all those in the

TABLE 55

Middle-grade medical workers in the USSR, USA and UK (rates per 10,000) for 1965

	USSR	USA	UK
Nurses	32·9	45·0*	39·0†
Feldshers and feldsher–midwives	20·5	2·0 (public health nurses)	5·5 (health visitors and medical social workers)
Midwives	7·4	—	10·5
Radiographers	0·9	3·6	1·0
Laboratory technicians	2·8	2·0	2·0
Pharmacists	5·5	6·0	5·0
Others	8·5	9·8	2·0
TOTAL	78·5	68·4	65·0

* Excluding 35 per 10,000 'aides' and 'orderlies'.
† Excluding 12 per 10,000 'other nurses'.

medical field. In order that realistic and reliable comparisons of utilisation may be made, careful and accurate work studies should be carried out – using comparable methods and techniques. Such studies could be carried out through the World Health Organisation.

A Personal Evaluation

Considerable differences exist in the present rates of medical manpower resources in all three countries and these differences are particularly notable when we consider physicians, the respective proportions being: USSR 1·9; USA 1·36; UK 1·00. Similar differences with some of the more specific types of middle-grade medical workers, Soviet feldshers being a special type which does not exist in either of the other countries.

Taking account of possible differences of nomenclature and definitions these differences indicate a need for the critical evaluation and assessment of role, function and the usage of medical manpower resources.

The increases in the numbers of physicians in the past 15 years (1950–1965) show that in the USSR the growth rate was 103 per cent, in the USA 34 per cent and in the UK 33 per cent, but recommendations have been made in all three nations that the output of medical graduates should be doubled in the next decade (UK: Royal Commission on Medical Education, 1968; USA: *Health Manpower Perspective 1967*; and plans quoted to WHO Seminar in USSR in 1967).

In view of the serious absence of detailed factual data in any depth on the utilisation of medical manpower resources it is doubtful if such massive expansions are justified.

The evolution of health teams in the community has been slow and no information on really large scale experiments is available, but it is highly suggestive from experiences in the UK that closer co-operation and collaboration between various members of the greater medical profession, with more delegation from physician to auxiliary, may lead to a reduced need for medical manpower.

Studies are urgently required to provide more facts on analysis of work being done by physicians and others, and more data is required on the efficiency of the methods being used and on the quality of results. Experiments are required into different methods of using medical resources to establish possible new roles and functions of the medical workers and the tools and supportive organisation required. Such studies should ideally be carried out jointly through the World Health Organisation. The ultimate question is: 'Do we simply need more new medical manpower, or can we do more with our existing resources?' – and so far none of the three countries has answered this question critically and satisfactorily.

Chapter 12
Education and Training

The quality of any nation's medical care depends to a great extent on the education and training of its medical and paramedical workers. The essence of a successful process of education must be a flexibility that is able to meet the challenge of new and changing patterns and techniques of care, and to keep pace with a medical technology that is constantly on the move.

Medical Education in the USSR

GENERAL EDUCATION

In the USSR school attendance is compulsory between 7 and 15 years of age. In addition many children commence their education before the age of 7 through attending nurseries and kindergartens. It is stated that in the USSR 75 per cent of children between 3 and 6 years of age attend kindergartens and 25 per cent between 1 and 3 years of age attend nurseries. Those children who are selected for higher academic and technical careers remain at school till 18 and then proceed to university or technical college.

PHYSICIANS

Undergraduate Period

There are 85 medical schools or institutes in the USSR, all are state owned and all have the same basic curriculum, organisation and administration. Most medical schools are not part of a university and are relatively independent, being responsible directly to the Ministry of Health.

The output of medical graduates in 1965 was 28,000 but it is intended to increase this to 40,000 by 1975. This means that in 1965 each medical school graduated a class of 330 physicians. Assuming that there will be no new medical schools, by 1975 the number of medical graduates per medical school will be 470. Approximately 65 per cent of graduating Soviet physicians are women.

Medicine is popular amongst young Soviet citizens and the number of applicants for each medical school place is between 6 and 15. Selection is on merit and certain personal qualifications. Academic merit is assessed through an entrance examination in physics, chemistry and russian. Priority is given to feldshers who have completed more than three years in their work and who wish to train as physicians and in some years up to 20–30 per cent of all new medical students have had experience as feldshers or in allied work.

Each medical school has three faculties – therapy (general medical subjects), paediatrics and hygiene (public health) and the new medical student has to select one of these faculties and be accepted into it. In this way there is control of the proportion of physicians in these three groups but the student has to decide, even before starting his course, whether to be a public health physician, paediatrician, or other specialist.

The standard curriculum is six years and for the first two years students who are feldshers may enrol as evening students, continuing with their regular work during the day.

Medical education, as all education in the USSR, is free and students also receive adequate grants to maintain themselves. The first three years are the same in the three faculties of therapy, paediatrics and hygiene. Years 1 and 2 are spent in studying human biology, anatomy, physiology, Latin, foreign languages, humanities and russian, the third year includes pathology and pharmacology, and the final two are in clinical subjects related to the chosen faculty.

The final year (6) is spent in specialised elective subjects and the students may work in polyclinics or hospital units.

Throughout the medical course the students are expected also to take part in extra-curricular social activities that are a contribution to the community, such as in youth movements and general social work. It is at the end of the sixth year, when students are 23–25 years old, that the final examination is taken. There is a low overall failure rate and 95 per cent of all students entering medical school eventually graduate as physicians.

General Professional Training

On qualification all physicians undergo a three-year period of civilian medical work, to which they are directed by the Ministry of Health. This direction of medical labour is accepted as a national service by the students and as a form of repayment to the State by the individual. The selection of appointments is made on the basis of individual quality, merit and ability, on personal choice and to a large degree on national needs and requirements. The top 5–10 per cent of students who have achieved excellence during their undergraduate period are selected for academic and research careers and are offered appointments in the best teaching and research units. Some 40 per cent of graduates are sent to rural and outlying areas to work under the supervision of more experienced colleagues. They receive special inducements such as extra pay and special allowances (e.g. free housing and cheap coal) for working in these less popular areas. The largest proportion (more than one-half) of graduates will work in urban hospitals and polyclinics on a rotating basis for their three years of directed service.

Further Specialist Training

The medical career structure and professional progression in the USSR are along established lines and depend on merit and hard work.

After the three years of directed service the young physician can choose one of seventy-five specialities in which to make a career, and this specialist programme is then of two forms.

The 'ordinants', with no serious ambitions, undertake a two-year specialist course which consists of a clinical training appointment together with a period at a postgraduate institute. They then become clinical specialists at polyclinics, hospitals or public health units, but are unlikely to become chiefs of their departments.

'Aspirants' are the more able and ambitious young physicians who seek a higher level clinical, research or academic career. Their course of specialist training extends over three years and includes clinical work, a research project and a thesis, with, at the end of this period an examination for the diploma of 'Candidate of Medical Science'. Professional specialist appointments are made by application and competition and selections made on merit, ability and experience. There is a 'grading' of specialists – 'super', 'first' and 'second', and each grade has its own level of pay, length of annual leave and authority. After 15–20 years in his specialist branch the physician may present a thesis based on his own original work and research and submit it for the award of a 'Doctorate in Medical Science'. Such a qualification assists in further progress in the academic field leading to professorship and possible eventual election as Academician of the USSR Academy of Medical Sciences, the highest professional body.

Continuing Postgraduate Education and Training

Regular continuing postgraduate studies are compulsory for all but the very top physicians, and even they are required to undergo a recognised course of training every 3–5 years.

These courses may be carried out at one of the thirteen postgraduate institutes (45,000 to 50,000 physicians attend these institutes each year) or at regional or district centres. As noted in Chapter 4, part of the training of polyclinic physicians is the regular exchange with physicians working in local district hospitals.

MIDDLE-GRADE MEDICAL WORKERS

The training of Soviet middle-grade medical workers is the responsibility of the Ministry of Health of the USSR. In 1965 there were 540 schools training a quarter of a million such workers. This means that with an annual output of 85,000–90,000 (two and three-year courses) qualified workers each year, each school has an annual class of 160–200 students. On entry the candidates are 15–17 years of age and have completed 8–10 years of normal schooling. For those who leave school at 15 years of age the course is three years and for those who leave school at 17 (after ten years of schooling) the length of course is two years.

The three-year course is as follows:

Year 1 (for those leaving school at 15–16). General subjects designed to bring the student's education up to a required level.

Year 2. General medicine, pathology and hygiene.

Year 3. Special subjects depending on the type of worker being trained (there are ten types such as nurses, feldshers, technicians, etc. (see Chapter 11)).

Auxiliaries who work with the middle-grade workers receive a practical in-service training of 1–3 years, and all middle-grade medical workers are required to attend courses of continuing education for three months every 3–5 years. A special feature of the feldsher category is that feldshers are encouraged to become physicians if they meet academic entry requirements to medical schools, thus 20–30 per cent of all medical students are ex-feldshers and every year 2–5 per cent of feldshers enter medical schools to become physicians.

Medical Education in the USA

GENERAL EDUCATION

School starts at the age of 6 in the USA, although many children are sent to private kindergartens at an earlier age. Most children attend public schools and colleges and from 6–14 years children attend Primary School, then they pass on to High School for four years. Those who wish to continue further education then attend College or University until the age of 22, when they graduate. In the case of medicine this is followed by a further four years' study in a medical school. University education is not free in the USA and is paid for by the student and his family or through a system of state loans which are repayable when the student graduates. (Approximately 40 per cent of medical students receive state loans for their education.)

PHYSICIANS

Undergraduate Period

There were 85 medical schools in the USA in 1965, and most of these were associated with universities – but there were 10 that were independent. In 1965 there were 7,500 physicians who graduated out of some 8,300 who started on their courses six years before, a figure that represents a 90 per cent 'graduation-rate' (*Health Manpower Perspective 1967*). Only 5 per cent of medical graduates are women.

The mean size of each annual class in the American medical school, in 1965, was 88 graduates. There are about 2 applicants for each place in medical schools and to be selected for entry students must have completed 3 or 4 years in college and preferably have achieved a degree in biology, chemistry and physics. There is no specialisation in the undergraduate period and a general curriculum is followed over a period of six years that covers basic medical sciences and clinical subjects. At the end of their period of training, successful students graduate as doctors of medicine (MD).

General Professional Training

Following qualification, all physicians now carry out one year as a hospital intern and then most follow this with a period of 2–5 years as a resident. The internship of one year is now considered as a preliminary to a residency, and is intended as the phase where the newly qualified graduate can begin to gain practical clinical experience under the close supervision of specialists and residents. This period of training is not under the control of universities or medical schools but the hospitals receiving interns have to be approved and accredited by a Joint Committee on Hospital Accreditation, on which serve representatives from the American Medical and Hospitals Associations and from College of Surgeons. Only 12 per cent of US community hospitals (600 out of 5,100) are accredited and thus able to attract junior medical staff.

At the end of the intern year (or later) the young physician is able to sit the local State Board Certificate which will allow him to practise within that state.

In the USA medical legislation and certification is the responsibility of each state, which has its own Certificate, although there are some reciprocities, and if the physician moves out of his state to another where no reciprocal arrangements exist, then he has to pass a further certification board.

Further Specialist Training

The residency appointments are the preliminary to specialisation and this scheme involves a 2–5 year period of training at a recognised and accredited hospital. Only 18 per cent (1,300 out of 7,200) of all US hospitals are recognised for residencies (*U.S.A. 1967*).

This training may be carried out completely under the personal supervision of the chief of Service of the particular hospital specialty, or a 'rotating residency' may be undertaken in a series of general departments. At the end of their 3–5 year residency period the potential specialist sits for a Specialty Board examination, which is designed to set the seal on completion of specialist training. These Boards are under the control and direction of elected members of a specialty and there are now twenty-six such different boards, each for a recognised medical specialty. In addition to examining candidates and issuing certificates, the Boards set the standards and the curricula to be followed, advise individuals on appropriate courses and ensure that adequate facilities exist in the accredited hospitals. Specialty Board Certification is now successfully achieved by 80 per cent of all medical graduates and the proportion is increasing each year. The possession of a board certificate is now being required as a criterion of suitability of a physician for facilities by more and more community hospitals. Following attainment of the specialty board certificate, and before entering independent practice, some physicians take a fellowship for one or two years to work in research or in a special field under the guidance of an eminent colleague.

Continuing Education

Continuing medical education and training is not compulsory in the USA but is nevertheless widely recognised as essential. There are many courses available for both first-contact physicians and specialists but according to A.G.W. Whitfield (*Lancet* (1963), *2*, 514) only one-quarter of all physicians in America attend postgraduate courses in any year and they tend to be the same group.

MIDDLE-GRADE MEDICAL WORKERS

Nurses

There are three possible courses of training for registered nurses.

1. Baccalaureate degree from a university – a course extending over 4–5 years.

2. A Diploma from a hospital Nursing School – 3 years.

3. An Associate Degree from a community college – 2 years.

In 1965 there were 35,000 new registered nurses from 1,200 schools, colleges and universities – an output of approximately 30 per school, and the proportions of the various groups were: Baccalaureates (16 per cent), Diplomates (77 per cent), and Associate degree holders (7 per cent).

During the same year 25,000 practical nurses were trained in recognised hospital schools or under the local public vocational school system. Other middle-grade medical groups are much fewer in numbers and have their own recognised courses of training lasting 1–3 years.

Medical Education in the UK

GENERAL EDUCATION

Schooling is compulsory in the United Kingdom between 5 and 15 years, and there is a free state education system from nursery school to postgraduate university studies. At the same time those parents who wish can send their children to private schools (approximately 15 per cent of children attend private schools). Between 5 and 11, children attend primary schools, and at 11 they may enter grammar (academic), technical or secondary modern schools, depending on their aptitudes. Comprehensive schools are a recent development in the system where all children between 11 and 18 attend a single school within which various courses may be organised for the child. Public schools are private academic and grammar schools for children between the ages of 13 and 19, where there is a mixture of fee-paying, scholarship and grant-aided pupils, and at many public schools the boys live as boarders and return home for holidays. These are old and traditional schools, the oldest being nearly 800 years old. At 17–18, school children take an examination in three or four selected subjects (the general certificate of education) and on their success in this examination depends whether they are admitted to university or other colleges of further education.

Education and Training

Undergraduate Period

Entry into one of the twenty-five medical schools depends on high-level passes in chemistry, physics and biology at the school examinations, and all the 25 medical schools are faculties of a university. Competition for places at medical schools is intense and there are between 3 and 6 applications for each place. In 1965 there were 12,000 medical students in the UK and of these 25 per cent were women. In 1965, there were 1,618 new medical graduates, a rate of 65 per each medical school. All British students accepted into medical schools receive state grants for fees, books, living expenses and travel.

The medical curriculum lasts 5 years, and the first 2 years are spent studying anatomy, physiology, pharmacology and biochemistry. At the end of this period an examination is taken. The second period of 3 years is spent in a teaching hospital of the medical school studying the various branches of medicine, hygiene and pathology, and at the end of these 5 years a qualifying examination (MB, BS) is taken and 92 per cent of all students eventually qualify.

The curriculum of all medical schools has to be approved by the General Medical Council, whose function it is to ensure the quality and ethics of medical practice.

General Professional Training

A period of one year in a recognised hospital pre-registration appointment is required before the new physician is allowed to become registered and practise independently. These appointments are usually in general medical and surgical specialities and are designed to add an extra year of compulsory training before full registration. Following this compulsory year most physicians work for a further two or three years in hospital appointments before undertaking a specialist training. There is no special organisation or direction into these appointments apart from meeting the requirements of any selected specialist qualifying examination and the selection is left entirely to the physician.

Further Specialist Training

Further training depends on the branch of medical care the physician chooses to follow.

For general practice there is as yet no definitive and recognised training, although it is recommended that prospective general practitioners undergo 3–5 years of post-registration training in hospital and general practice, but at present there are few courses available and because of a relative shortage young physicians can obtain appointments in general practice without any special training.

For public health practice, physicians obtain a Diploma in Public Health (DPH) and have to have had some 5–10 years of experience in this field in junior positions before being appointed to a senior grade.

For hospital practice, there is a more definitive course of postgraduate training, with 5–10 years as a 'registrar', in recognised hospital appointments, being required before the physician is eligible for appointment as a consultant specialist in the National Health Service. During this period he is expected to have passed one or more of the many postgraduate specialist diplomas and degrees as a sign of his ability. These diplomas may be Fellowship of the Royal College of Surgeons (FRCS), Membership of the Royal College of Physicians (MRCP), Membership of the Royal College of Obstetricians and Gynaecologists (MRCOG) or the degrees of Doctor of Medicine (MD), or Master of Surgery (MS). (These are all difficult examinations with pass rates of only 20–40 per cent.)

Once appointed as Consultant in the National Health Service the specialist is not specifically required to undertake any further training.

Continuing Education and Training

It is chiefly in the field of general practice that most continuing education is carried out, and there are many courses available at universities and at all of 200 medical centres based on district hospitals. Under the National Health Service general practitioners are allowed generous fees and expenses for attending recognised courses and in 1965 nearly 60 per cent attended such courses.

Education and Training

The training periods for the main middle-grade workers, namely, nurses and associates, are as follows:

Nurses. State Registered Nurses (SRN) three years' hospital course. State Enrolled Nurses (SEN) two years' practical training in hospital.

Midwives have to be SRN nurses and they then carry out a further one year of training in two parts of six months. The first part is hospital-based and the second six months is carried out in the community services, and at the end of this year an examination is carried out and successful candidates become State Certified Midwives (SCM).

Health Visitors are SRN nurses who have also carried out some or all of the midwifery course (SCM), and fulfilled a further year of extra training so that her total time in training is five years.

Some Comparisons of Medical Education

There is a striking similarity in the systems of medical education in all three countries.

The total length of undergraduate training is similar, between five and six years; the courses are divided into comparable stages and the graduate and postgraduate further education is also on similar patterns.

GENERAL EDUCATION

The whole picture of the educational process from school to medical graduation in each nation is shown in Fig. 13, and again there is not a great deal of difference. The total periods from starting school to medical graduation are 17 years in the USSR, 20 years in the USA, and 18 years in the UK. Schooling lasts 11, 12 and 13 years respectively and the age of starting school is 7 years in the USSR, 6 in the USA and 5 in the UK. At school the primary and secondary stages are carried out at different establishments with the change-over taking place at 11 years in the USSR and the UK, and at 14 in the USA. Entry into university (or college in USA) is at 18 in all three systems.

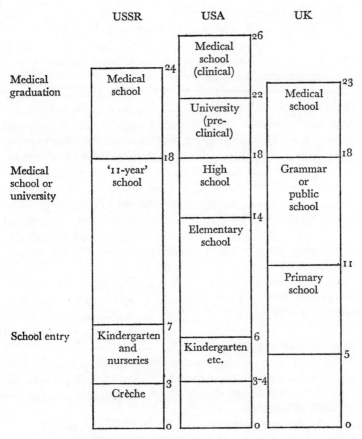

Fig. 13. General school education in the USSR, the USA and the UK. (Ages in years.)

PHYSICIANS

Undergraduate Period

There is an excess of demand for places in the medical schools in all three nations, and Medicine is obviously a popular profession. All applicants have to achieve certain comparable entrance standards, based on examination results, and final selection has to be made on individual criteria and qualities, on the basis of further tests and interviews.

221

The pre-clinical and clinical courses are similar but the major difference is that the Soviet medical student has to select one of three special faculties at the start of his training, whereas in the USA and the UK there is a common system of education for all medical students.

The Americans have a more definite demarcation between pre-clinical and clinical periods. The pre-clinical course is a three or four-year degree course at college or university, at the end of which the student is awarded a BA (Bachelor of Arts) degree. He then enters medical school as a graduate for a four-year clinical course.

In the UK there is a choice for students. The majority take a set five-year degree course for MB, BS (Bachelor of Medicine and Bachelor of Surgery), but a minority take an extra year in the pre-clinical period, to complete a three-year course for the BSc (Bachelor of Science) degree and follow this by three years of clinical studies.

Although the general pattern and context of the medical curriculum are the same in the three systems, differences of detail and emphasis exist. For example there is more emphasis in the Soviet system on prevention, hygiene and military medicine. In the USA and the UK individual medical schools are able to develop their own programmes, with wide variations, providing that overall curricula meet statutory requirements.

Table 56 sets out various comparable data on the numbers of medical schools and students in the three countries.

The factor that stands out in the table of comparisons is the ability of the USSR to cope with large numbers of students, most of whom are females. The annual rate per 100,000 of the population of medical graduations is more than three times that of the USA and four times that of the UK. Associated with this is the large size of each annual class in the 85 Soviet medical schools, for in 1965 the average size of class was 330 students, compared with averages of 88 in the USA and 64 in the UK.

This ability to deal with large numbers of students is a feature of the whole Soviet system of education, also noted by John Vaizey in *Education in the Modern World* (London, 1967) who states that "perhaps the most extraordinary feature of the (Soviet) system has been its success in coping

TABLE 56

Some comparable data on medical education

	USSR	USA	UK
Populations (millions)	230	200	50
Number of medical schools	85	85	25
Age of entry	18	18 (or 22 if pre-clinical course at college)	18
Applicants per place at medical school	Between 5 and 15 depending on school	2	5–6
Length of curriculum (years)	6	8 (4 years pre-clinical and 4 years clinical)	5 or 6
Annual class per medical school	330	88	64
Annual numbers of graduates (1965)	28,000	7,500	1,600
Annual rate of medical graduates per 100,000 of population	12·2	3·75	3·2
Graduation rates for all students who start on medical course	95 per cent	90 per cent	90 per cent
Percentage of female medical students	65 per cent	5 per cent	25 per cent

with huge numbers. The child population has doubled since the Revolution and the number of children at school has multiplied many more times. The number of teachers per child is the highest in the world and the output of Soviet universities and technical institutions rivals that of the United States. . . . Perhaps the most distinctive feature of Soviet education has been the way in which expanson has been controlled and centrally developed while at the same time releasing local support and initiative."

Graduate and Postgraduate Education

Immediately after qualification the young physicians in the three nations work in recognised and approved training appointments under the supervision of senior colleagues. In the USA and the UK this compulsory period of internship or pre-registration is one year and the choice of the place and nature of the appointment is left to the physician. In the USSR there is a compulsory period of three years of national service where the physician is sent to the places where the need for medical services is greatest.

Further general and specialist training programmes are similar – for the budding specialists there are 3–5 years of hard work in preparation of special examinations, the "Candidate of Medical Science" in the USSR, the "Specialty Board Certificate" in the USA and the "Membership" and "Fellowship" of either the Royal College of Physicians or Surgeons, in the UK. However it is interesting to note that whilst continuing education is compulsory for all physicians in the USSR, it is merely 'strongly recommended' in the USA and the UK.

MIDDLE-GRADE MEDICAL WORKERS

The multiple subdivisions in this field make comparison difficult but as far as nurses are concerned, and these are the largest group in the greater medical profession, the basic training periods are similar. The Soviet nurse and feldsher has a three-year curriculum; in the USA the period of training ranges from four years for a nursing degree course, through three years for a diploma and two years for an associate degree; and in the UK the period of training for state registration is three years, with extra periods of one year for midwifery and a further year for health visitors.

Table 57 shows some comparative data for nurse training.

The proportion of nurses being trained is highest in the UK, but particularly notable is the large size of class in the Soviet schools of nursing.

A Personal Evaluation

It has been accepted that medical education is a life-long process, comprising well recognised phases, which require special arrangements and organisation. It is acknowledged also that the purpose of training must be to fit the medical

TABLE 57

Nurse training in the USSR, the USA and the UK

	USSR	USA	UK
Period of nursing training (years)	3–3½ for nurses and feldshers	4 for nursing degree 3 for nursing diploma 2 for associate nursing degree	3 for state registered nurse 4 for midwife 5 for health visitor
Annual output of all new nurses	88,000	60,000 (35,000 registered nurses, 25,000 practical nurses)	27,000 (17,500 SRN 7,500 SEN 2,000 midwives)
Annual rates of new nurses per 100,000	38	30	50
Average numbers per class in nursing school	175	30	15

worker for the role and responsibilities that he, or she, is to undertake in the health services. Since the forms of medical care are changing so medical training must be sufficiently flexible to meet changes and experiments. In large national systems of education such flexibility requires considerable decentralisation and freedom of action for local schools, but at the same time central co-ordination is required to apply the results.

Specialisation is an inevitable trend. In the USSR all physicians are considered specialists, and in the USA four out of every five medical graduates achieve specialty board certification. In the UK the recent Royal Commission on Medical Education (1968, London) recommends that "all doctors – general practitioners as well as consultants – will be specialists in particular aspects of medicine who will be equally regarded as such and will be fully trained for the work they undertake". Therefore there has to be a special period of vocational specialist training for all physicians.

A feature of the Soviet medical education system is the large number of graduates being produced and the large size of the annual classes at each medical school. It is possible that such large schools are more efficient than those with less than 100 graduates each year which are found in the USA and the UK. The Royal Commission on Medical Education has also recommended that all British medical schools treble their annual output to at least 200 graduates a year.

The training of middle-grade medical workers is unsettled because the roles that these workers may carry out are uncertain and changing. The example of the work of the feldsher in the Soviet system has demonstrated some of the possibilities of such workers working alongside and in collaboration with physicians. If their successful example is to be followed then special training courses may have to be devised in the USA and the UK.

It is urgent that a complete re-examination of the roles and functions of all who work in the 'greater medical profession' is made, in order that changes in training can be brought about to equip them for providing the medical care of the future. Any such re-examination should include an international comparison of role, function, nomenclature and training programmes.

Chapter 13
The Present Dilemmas of Medical Care

A CHANGING WORLD

There is a changing public attitude to health, disease and care. It is a much more educated public – educated not only through better schooling and vocational and technical training, but also through the modern mass media of communication of the press, radio and television. It is a more expectant and a less tolerant public. Expectant of service and a high quality of care. In a scientific and technological era it often expects what may be medically impossible and is less tolerant of failures and mistakes. In a personal sense the individual is less prepared to tolerate sickness and discomfort and expects modern medical science to relieve and comfort him always, even if he can be cured only sometimes.

Scientific advances are apparently limitless in a world of space travel, computer innovations and nuclear science and many of these newly found techniques have been applied to medical care and have radically altered both its scope and its opportunities.

Within medicine the old 'killer' diseases associated with ignorance, poverty and dirt are being rapidly controlled, only to be replaced by the modern disorders associated with affluence and self-neglect. Although most of us will live longer, not many will live beyond the allotted span of "three-score years and ten".

With the scientific and technological advances there has

been a knowledge explosion that has brought with it a rapid growth and development of specialisation within medicine. It has been assumed, often erroneously, that no one man can work alone in his field and that therefore all physicians must become 'specialists'. The problem is over the definition of 'specialist' and the dangers of specialisation in neglecting humane care of the sick as individuals and family groups. In this changing world there is no single national system of medical care that can be applied to every nation but there are certain principles within national systems that can and should be applicable to others.

COMMON DILEMMAS

In all nations attempts are being made to provide maximum health at minimum cost, but this is increasingly difficult. Particular difficulties are encountered with increasing costs, and the cost of medical care in the USA and the UK (noted in Chapter 3) and the proportions of gross national product being spent on medical care, are steadily increasing.

How high should these costs be allowed to rise is a problem facing all developed societies, for it seems that the proportion of GNP alloted to health and medical services is related to social advancement. Medical care can easily become a bottomless pit, and with the 'vacuum of sophistication' and the 'mirage of health' controls must be exercised.

Another problem, in some ways more difficult to resolve, is the relative shortage of skilled medical manpower that is occurring in developed societies. This arises not only because of the need for more physicians and nurses but because of increasing competition for high quality students from other professions. So far this problem is not apparent in the three nations under review for applications for medical places still outnumber available places, but in the USA and the UK there are real shortages of nurses.

In most nations it is inevitable that there will always be a deficiency of medical resources to meet all needs and wants. Decisions will have to be taken therefore and policies made to arrive at priorities to introduce some scheme of rationing, and to arrive at some means or needs tests involving 'gate keepers' or 'controllers' whereby available resources can be allocated fairly and with justice.

EFFICIENT UTILISATION OF RESOURCES

With an increasing demand on available resources it is important that they should be used efficiently and effectively, but unfortunately the application to medical care of modern methods and techniques of business efficiency and work analysis has been slow, because of understandable fundamental problems. Firstly there are basic difficulties in collecting the factual data that is required, in order to make a reasonable analysis of existing situations, but then even greater human and material difficulties arise in attempts to change faulty techniques and methods that are uncovered.

The operational data that ought to be constantly collected might be as follows:

1. The existing state of morbidity and mortality, including whenever possible the extent of undiagnosed and untreated social and medical disorders in the community.
2. The work load carried by the 'greater medical profession' in dealing with the existing morbidity, that presents for care.
3. The methods and techniques of care employed by the medical profession, which must then be analysed critically to determine whether maximal utilisation of resources is being achieved.
4. Some qualitative measures and indices must be included to take note of the outcome of the care given, and of the satisfaction that it gives to the consumers, and to the standards of the profession.

Before any findings of collected data can be applied, there must be a stage of experiment and evaluation. There are no examples of such planned experiments in medical care in any of the three systems described. Nor is there any practical and reliable data on which useful international comparisons can be made – comparability at present is impossible because data collected from all countries arises from differing definitions and criteria.

When it comes to the application of operational data the following problems occur:

1. Professional freedom, independence and autonomy are praiseworthy and justifiable, because a servile and over-

controlled profession cannot produce the best system of medical care. Within the context of professional autonomy there must evolve a responsible leadership through which new ideas and methods of care can be introduced.

2. State interest and subsidisation of medical care must inevitably lead to controls, directives and national planning of medical and social services. Some compromise will have to be achieved between the profession and the state.

3. The system of care must be flexible and amenable to change. This flexibility should include the attitudes of the public and profession as well as the design of buildings and the conduct of any general administration.

THE SYSTEM

There is agreement that wherever possible medical care by well-qualified physicians and aides should be available and accessible to all, but differences exist between the nations in the ways in which this is paid for.

It is accepted generally that the costs of total medical care are now out of reach of the private individual's pocket and beyond the means of private insurance. Total medical care that includes personal care from physicians and hospitalisation for all illnesses; preventive measures and health education; public health services including safe food and water, clean air, sanitation and hygiene; and various complementary social and welfare services – no private or semi-public organisation can possibly pay for all such services.

A number of different methods have been developed to pay for medical care, but in the end it is the individual who pays for it either directly of indirectly. Whether he pays partly out of his own pocket, or through pre-paid insurance, or through direct taxation, or through the costs being taken by the state at source, it is still the citizens of any country who pay.

There are other details to be considered. Should the patient pay at the time of service in order to give him a sense of personal responsibility? Should he then be reimbursed for most of what he has paid the physician from the state or insurance company? Should the physician be paid fees for services, on a capitation basis or by salary?

The national systems of Soviet Russia, America and the United Kingdom offer three possibilities – there are many more possible variations. The question that demands an answer is – does the system of payment, finance and budgeting make any real difference to the final quality of care?

Thus, in the Soviet system the financing is done at source. With no system of taxation it is agreed that some 7 per cent of the total budget be set aside for medical care. The Soviet citizen receives free medical care (apart from certain exceptions for which nominal payments are made, i.e. drugs, appliances, dentures and legal abortions). The Soviet physicians and other medical workers are paid by agreed salary scales. Capital and maintenance costs are all budgeted for from central sources.

In the American system the emphasis is on personal responsibilities for medical care with a free-enterprise scheme of private care for those who can pay for it. However, it has proved impossible for such a scheme, that includes pre-paid insurance and participation from employers, big business organisations and trade unions as well as private individuals, to meet all costs. The federal and state governments also have to provide considerable (see Chapter 3) proportions of facilities and costs of medical care in the USA.

The British system with the National Health Service is paid for in a mixture of ways. Some of the costs come from pre-paid insurance by employees and employers and some from direct payments for prescriptions and dental care, but most of the costs come from direct taxation (see Chapter 3).

Which system is the best? It is impossible to say. Physicians seem most satisfied in the American system and patients least satisfied. Some physicians appear very unhappy under the Britsh system, but more than 90 per cent of the public on repeated enquiries say they are well satisfied. As far as an outside observer can judge, the Soviet system is acceptable equally to profession and consumers. As for qualitative indices, it is doubtful whether the form of system has made any ultimate difference to the health of Soviet, American or British citizens.

ADMINISTRATIVE LEVELS

All systems of medical care must have administrative levels

of organisation which must be related to population size and local geography.

The following are administrative units that appear practical in most systems.

1. *National level* represents the overall planning and policy-making body – the Ministry or a Department of Health within a broader Ministry.
2. *State or Republic level.* In nations of great size such as the USSR or the USA, a State (one of fifty in the USA) or a Republic (one of thirteen in the USSR) have considerable autonomy and independence of action.
3. *Region* (500,000–5 million). In most nations the administrative level immediately after the top national unit is the region (or *'oblast'* in the USSR).With populations of from 500,000 to 5 million to administer, the functions of the regional medical care unit are to supervise the lower district levels and to arrange for regional hospitals with many of the super-specialist units such as chest and heart surgical units, neurological and neurosurgical centres, radiotherapy units with cobalt-bomb or other very expensive apparatus.

   In the USSR with its highly planned hospital system the *'oblast'* (regional) hospital is able to function as a super-specialist centre. It does not admit cases direct from the community but only through special referral from district hospitals. The chiefs of the more general specialties such as medicine, surgery and gynaecology–obstetrics, have the added responsibilities of ensuring a high quality of care in their respective specialities within the whole region. They are involved with the continuing training of specialists, with promotions, with visiting outlying hospitals and with organising specialist teams or groups available to visit other hospitals or centres to give their opinions and advice or to assist in complex therapeutic procedures.
4. *District* (50,000–500,000). A district is a population and geographical unit of a size justifiably served by a district or community hospital that can provide the general and customary specialist hospital services. The size will depend on the type of area. Thus a district hospital will include general medical, surgical and gynaecological–obstetric

departments, with other visiting specialists such as ophthalmology, ear, nose and throat, dermatology, orthopaedics and psychiatry. Admissions for these latter specialities may be into the district hospital or to some other regional centres.

Facilities for ambulant specialist services will be provided either at the district hospital or in polyclinics or other centres. Ideally, the district medical services should work as a single unit combining hospital, public health and first-contact services with a single administration. This has been achieved in the USSR where the Chief Physician of the District is responsible for all the medical services.

5. *Neighbourhood–Locality* (500–50,000). The most peripheral administrative division of medical care services is the neighbourhood or locality. In a densely populated and flat-dwelling urban community, a neighbourhood population of 50,000 may be cared for easily from a single medical (or health) centre as demonstrated in the USSR polyclinics and in US medical groups. Such centres can provide social, welfare, health educational and other paramedical facilities in addition to traditional medical care. In rural areas a different system is necessary and the Soviet pattern is a good example.

There, as described in Chapter 4, the centre is the rural (neighbourhood) polyclinic–hospital where the main medical resources are based. Associated with this centre and responsible to its physicians are a series of feldsher–midwife (medical aid) posts staffed by specially trained paramedical middle-grade medical workers. The population served by each rural polyclinic–hospital may be 5,000–20,000, but a feldsher–midwife post may serve a population of only 500.

LEVELS OF CARE

Just as there are particular levels of administration in the organisation of medical care, so there are more personal levels in the flow of care to those who are sick and in need.

In Chapters 4, 5 and 6, the first-contact, specialist ambulatory and hospital services have been described and now they are reconsidered in order to examine future trends.

Q*

The Present Dilemmas of Medical Care

The Family

The 'family' group is accepted now as the basic social unit. This being so it is necessary to consider whether 'family care' is a reasonable proposition, but whether this care is provided by a single 'family doctor', by a single group of specialists or by a team that includes paramedical workers is immaterial. These and other forms of family care can be organised readily if there is a general agreement and desire to provide care for the family as a single unit. It is only in the UK that there is any evidence of such family care being attempted, and here it is largely the result of a National Health Service that perpetuated pre-existing and traditional patterns of organisation.

In the USSR and the USA the philosophy of specialisation has been accepted and this has prevented the development of any general scheme for the care of families as single units. It is customary in Soviet cities for each member of the family to attend different physicians and in the USA a similar pattern has emerged.

There is not enough evidence to decide which system is the better one, but it is appropriate that the question be examined further not only from the purely medical aspect but also from a sociological point of view.

Family Responsibilities

The individual and the family have certain responsibilities in the maintenance of health and prevention of disease. Much is known now of the causes of disease and there are specific preventive measures that can be taken. Implementation depends largel yon individual action and co-operation. Cigarette smoking is a major causal factor in cancer of the lung and lack of exercise and over-eating are associated with coronary heart disease. How far should individual responsibilities be pushed? Should reliance be placed on the nebulous hopes of health education or on the growth of screening clinics or should some more forceful methods be used, such as the principle of 'health activists' in the USSR?

First-contact Care

The feature of first-contact care is that the local primary physician is the first person to be consulted by the patient and to whom the patient has direct access. He can, however, only care for a small neighbourhood population, and if this tends to be fairly static, then long-term and continuing care is a feature. Minor disease predominates. The primary physician has to act as an assessor, early diagnostician and co-ordinator of the whole system of local care.

With this closely defined role, one should consider whether it should be the single portal of entry to the medical care system as in the UK, or should there be a free choice for the patient to select the type of specialist or unit to attend? If he is considered as a family physician, well trained and organised to act as a co-ordinator of the medical services, then it is the best for the system that access to other levels is channelled through him, and he is responsible ultimately for his patients' long-term care. If it is considered that specialisation is of importance and that the public should be allowed the choice of specialist appropriate to their own interpretation of presenting symptoms, then there have to be a series of specialoids acting as primary physicians.

Whatever any society decides it should be pointed out that opportunities for clinical specialisation in any depth, at first-contact-care level, are, limited because of the nature of the material that the physician encounters.

What is obvious is that the days of the single-handed physician or the over-restricted group are over. Work in this field requires a team of physicians, nurses, social workers and others, just as much as does the work in hospitals.

The success of the Soviet feldsher in the rural areas and the satisfactory associations between general practitioners and nurses and health visitors in the UK shows that the concept of a health team at this level can lead to a more effective use of available resources. Whatever the system and the pattern of care, difficulties are now being experienced in attracting young physicians into this field of practice and in particular to rural and socially less desirable districts. Whilst some may protest against the direction of young Soviet physicians during their first three postgraduate years, it is a form of national service by which the individual repays the state for a free professional training.

A high standard of care can be attained only if there are adequate modern diagnostic and therapeutic facilities. The question of whether primary physicians should have direct access to hospital beds and full responsibility for treating their patients is unresolved. In the USA many primary physicians treat their patients in hospitals, but not in the other two countries. Whilst close association between primary physicians and hospitals is desirable, too much freedom to undertake complex clinical care is probably undesirable.

Specialist Care for Ambulatory Patients

A specialist service for ambulatory cases is necessary in all systems even when first-contact care is undertaken by 'specialists'. Such a specialist service acts in support of primary physicians, to which they may refer their problems. Features of such a service are physicians more highly trained in specific specialties, to whom cases are referred selectively and under whose care come populations that are much larger than those of primary physicians.

Under the Soviet and American systems patients have direct access to specialists; in contrast to the British NHS they are 'referred' by their general practitioners. The crux of the matter is one of continuing responsibility and care. Is the specialist to whom the patient has taken himself prepared to undertake continuing care and, if not, who is? In the USA the specialist undertakes the role of a physician of first contact and in the USSR the specialist may continue long-term care or refer the case back to the local therapist. However, it should not be assumed that ambulatory specialist services must be hospital based. In the USSR they are sited in the polyclinics and polyclinic specialists do not have access to hospital beds, whilst in the USA most specialists work from private rooms, groups or clinics that are geographically separate from hospitals. Whatever the place of consultation it seems highly desirable that specialists should have opportunities to treat these ambulatory patients when they are admitted to hospital.

Hospitals

Modern hospitals offer the most expert and most expensive care and they should therefore be used efficiently and economically. They should be planned and organised in a functional manner, ranging from small rural hospitals, through district, regional and university hospitals. The planning of hospitals should be on a national, regional and district basis with avoidance of competition and overlap and with high indices of utilisation and avoidance of over-long waiting lists.

Supportive Services

Supporting all these levels of care are the public health, welfare and social services, that in any good modern system of medical care should be integrated closely with the clinical and personal services.

Appendix
A Profile of District Medical Care

Faced with a hypothetical situation of planning for a modern urban district of 200,000 persons what can be distilled from the experiences gained by a study of the three systems of medical care?

THE SYSTEM

Any national system of medical care must be based on, and develop from, the national, cultural, political and economic philosophies of that country. Having accepted national influence, the system of medical care should be a single system planned, administered and organised for maximal effective utilisation. Within such a system there will have to be some degree of state and community involvement through the subsidisation of the mounting costs of care; there will have to be co-operation and collaboration from a medical profession that is prepared to acknowledge the inevitability of some restrictive controls for the sake of efficiency, but which also must retain considerable professional independence and autonomy; and certain recognised responsibilities will have to be accepted and undertaken by families and individuals if the system is to function well.

ADMINISTRATION

There should be a recognisable administrative framework that corresponds to the national administration, and at each level there should be active participation of community and professional representatives, and co-operation with skilled administrators.

A Profile of District Medical Care

At the national level decisions will be made on policies relating to overall budgeting and planning of resources. The regional level will represent the apex of a pyramid of care (Table 58) with the chief specialist, hospital, academic, operational-intelligence, public health and social and welfare units. The heads of the clinical units at the chief regional hospital will also have the responsibility of overseeing the provision of services in their specialty within the region and ensuring a high quality of care, and so in a corresponding way will the heads of the public health and social and welfare divisions.

TABLE 58

Regional and district structure of medical services

	Population	Functions	Activities
Regional	500,000–5 million	1. Super-specialist care for medical, public health and welfare.	1. Regional hospital with super-specialist units.
		2. Overall control and administration of regional services.	2. Super-specialist public health and social and welfare units.
		3. Education, training and research.	3. Regional administrative centre.
District	50,000–500,000	1. General specialist medical, public health and welfare services.	1. District hospital.
		2. Single administrative unit for all services.	2. Specialist services (medical, social, and welfare) for ambulatory.
		3. Local medical centre for training and research.	3. District administrative centre.

TABLE 58—*cont.*

	Population	Functions	Activities
Neighbourhood – locality	500–50,000	1. First contact primary personal care for medical, public health, social and welfare services	1. Community medical centre.
		2. Single community centre for all services.	2. Health Team care for families and individuals.
			3. Local administrative unit.

The district level will be concerned with the supply of personal and public health services for the standard diseases that are encountered in hospital and first-contact community practice.

A BLUEPRINT

Our hypothetical modern and urban district of 200,000 persons will be the administrative responsibility of a single chief district medical officer. He will be responsible for all the medical services in his district, including hospitals, public health facilities and primary medical and social services. Within this population of 200,000 there will be probably between 50,000 and 60,000 family units, and accepting the importance of the family as the basic social unit, family care should be provided.

First-contact care will be provided therefore from local medical centres and in a modern urban community there is a strong case for making the local neighbourhood units much larger than the customary 4,000 of the Soviet *uchastok*. Local medical centres should be planned to serve from 20,000 to 50,000 persons. In this way they will provide centralisation not only of primary medical services but also the local base for welfare and social security services. There will be, therefore, up to ten such local medical centres in our district with good diagnostic and therapeutic facilities for the care of the more common diseases, and each centre will be staffed by physicians and paramedical workers.

In my opinion there is at present an over-generous physician staffing of the first-contact services in all three countries. Experience in the UK and Sweden suggests that with more collaboration between physicians and paramedical workers it is possible to provide good medical care with fewer physicians for any defined size of population. It is quite feasible to consider a ratio of one primary physician to 4,000 persons, if he is a generalist, and that means that five primary physicians (of first contact) will be needed to staff a local medical centre serving an urban population of 20,000 However, if there is specialisation at this level into paediatric and general medical (internists) 'specialoids,' then this population will require probably two such paediatricians (1 : 2,000 children) and four internists (1 : 4,000 adults). These five or six physicians will be assisted by a team of middle-grade medical workers, nurses and clerical assistants, and for a centre serving 20,000 persons the following is a likely complement of paramedical staff:

Nurses	5–6 (1 per physician)
Medical social workers	2
Technicians	2
Clerical and secretarial	7
Manager	1

Considerable delegation of work is possible by physicians, providing that the paramedical workers are trained suitably and that the physician retains final responsibility. With five or six physicians the patients should be allowed free choice of physician and it should be possible also for them to select physicians working from other centres, providing that the distance is not too great.

The centre should provide facilities whereby specialists from the local district hospital can see patients referred to them, as consultants. by the primary physicians. In addition to their work at the local medical centre the primary physicians should be encouraged to work at the district hospital. This does not imply that they should carry out hospital care for all their patients, but that they should be attached to hospital departments as associates with regular sessions and responsibilities. If these sessions are numerous then the physician staffing of the centre will have to be correspondingly increased. These hospital attachments are important more as continuing educational exercises, than to give primary physicians the opportunities for hospital care of their patients.

Specialist staff in the district should not be separated into hospital and ambulatory. It is best if the same specialist covers both areas. The out-patient service of the district hospital for ambulatory patients could be provided through regular sessions by specialists at the local medical centre and at a central out-patient department at the hospital. The numbers of specialists required for a population of 200,000, based on the UK rates, could be as follows:

General physicians	3	(Each one with cardiological or respiratory or other special interests)
General surgeons	3	
Obstetrician gynaecologists	3	
Psychiatrists	2	
Paediatrician	1	
Geriatrician	1	
Ear, nose and throat specialist	1–2	
Eye specialist	1–2	
Orthopaedic surgeon	1–2	
Skin specialist	1	
TOTAL	17–20	(With others such as neurologists, cardiologists, etc., visiting when necessary)

This consulting specialist staff will be supported by 25–35 junior hospital trainee physicians.

The size of the district hospital will depend on whether there is to be one single hospital, whether there are to be separate hospitals for certain diseases such as tuberculosis, mental illness, etc., and on the size of the more specialised regional hospitals. Assuming that 10 hospital beds per 1,000 are to be required and supposing that there will be a large regional hospital centre of 5,000 beds serving 25 districts of 200,000 in a region of 5 million, then each district would be allocated 1,800 hospital beds. Ideally, these 1,800 beds should be centralised in a single 'balanced hospital community' that includes care for the long-stay the mentally sick and other chronic illnesses. Such a large single district hospital will have one of the local medical centres in its grounds and will have the opportunity also of acting as the local medical centre for educational and other professional purposes.

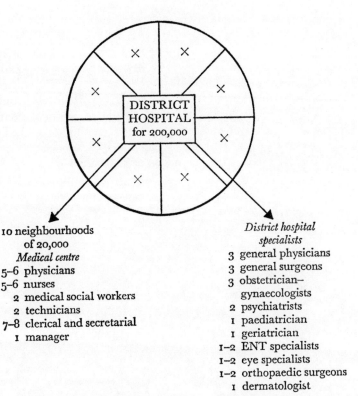

10 neighbourhoods
   of 20,000
   Medical centre
5–6 physicians
5–6 nurses
   2 medical social workers
   2 technicians
7–8 clerical and secretarial
   1 manager

*District hospital
   specialists*
3 general physicians
3 general surgeons
3 obstetrician–
   gynaecologists
2 psychiatrists
1 paediatrician
1 geriatrician
1–2 ENT specialists
1–2 eye specialists
1–2 orthopaedic surgeons
1 dermatologist

Fig. 14. Blueprint for District Medical Care.

Index

Index

Index